The

SHASTA PRESS

Candida Free Cookbook

125

**RECIPES TO
BEAT CANDIDA
AND LIVE
YEAST FREE**

CONTENTS

INTRODUCTION

This book is designed specifically for individuals who suffer from candida. As anyone who has been touched by candida knows, living with candida can change your life. The goal of this book is to help you change it again and take your health back.

Maybe you or someone close to you has been struggling with a variety of health problems for so long that you or that person has reached a breaking point. Maybe you don't even want to visit a doctor to describe your symptoms anymore, since you feel crazy trying to tell someone what's wrong. You aren't alone.

Here you will find all the facts you need and sound reasoning for the candida cleanse and diet. You will also find easy, delicious recipes that will help you relieve the symptoms of candida. The candida cleanse is a strict regimen, but it will help you and those you love who suffer with candida cope with the most severe symptoms.

Once you understand the way candida works in your body, the cleanse will make so much sense to you. This book will take you far beyond the simple cleanse. The candida diet is a long-term plan for living candida-free, and when you see and taste how good your meals can be while you feel your health improve, you will have the strength to complete the cleanse and change your routine for good.

Here is how the meal program works. The plan is broken down day by day, each described in detail, Day 1 through Day 14. Each day includes breakfast, a midmorning snack, lunch, a midday snack, dinner, and even a dessert. You will never go hungry. Many of the listed recipes are included in this book; these are denoted with asterisks.

More important, though, the basic principles of eating to beat candida are the nuts and bolts of this book. This means that you will soon have the tools to shape your own menus and meal plans, giving yourself both the freedom to eat how you please and the right foods to maintain your health.

One final note as you begin. If ever you have a bad day and go off your cleanse, just like anything else worth doing, try, try again. Your reasons for doing this cleanse and attempting to change your diet aren't just to lose a few pounds, for example. The improvement in your health that you can experience has the potential to be so much more profound.

Everyone makes a misstep here and there. If you do, don't beat yourself up. Just follow the tips provided here and you will have everything you need. In fact, keep your eyes peeled for little hints and tricks that will help you—whether you're soaring or struggling.

P A R T 1

Understanding Candida

1

WHAT IS CANDIDA?

If you are reading this book, chances are you already have an idea of what candida is, because you live with some constellation of symptoms every day. Even so, it is important to understand exactly what it is, what causes it, and what range of ailments can fall under the name "candida."

Candida itself is a fungus, a genus of yeast. *Candida albicans* is the most common species seen in humans. Because it plays a crucial role in digestion and nutrient absorption, it occurs naturally in your body. Normal amounts of candida include a very small amount of it in your mouth and somewhat more in your intestines. Unfortunately, candida can be overproduced, and that's the problem that this book addresses.

Candidiasis, also called thrush or a yeast infection, is an infection caused by candida. Candidiasis is also known to doctors as candidosis, moniliasis, and oidiomycosis. It is important to know that while candidiasis can be as simple as the thrush commonly seen in infants or the mild vaginal yeast infections seen in women, it can also be life-threatening. More serious infections are called candidemia, and usually they are seen in people who are severely immunocompromised, such as people with AIDS and cancer, or those healing from organ transplants and emergency surgeries.

Even milder cases of compromised immune systems allow candida to thrive more readily, however. For example, those with chronic fatigue syndrome (CFS)—at least one million Americans, according to experts—are more susceptible to infections, including candida infections. There are also many other ways that people can become vulnerable to candida symptoms.

Candida requires moisture to thrive. In terms of vaginal and colonic growth, there are multiple risk factors. Some of these include use of douches and other detergents, hormonal fluctuations that disturb the normal vaginal flora (including pregnancy, hormone replacement therapy, infertility treatment, and use of birth control pills), use of antibiotics that also kill off healthy vaginal flora, diabetes mellitus, and even wearing wet swimwear for extended periods of time.

Diet is also linked to rates of candida growth. Specifically, diets high in simple carbohydrates are great for candida and bad for people who suffer from overgrowth of candida.

Traditional medical doctors generally diagnose candidiasis using microscopic examination, culturing, or both methods in tandem. Treatments generally include antifungal drugs, also known as antimycotics. The most commonly prescribed drugs are fluconazole (usually taken orally), and the topical drugs clotrimazole, ketoconazole, and nystatin. Unfortunately, candida can develop resistance to fluconazole, which is currently the most effective drug. For seriously ill patients who develop resistance, such as those with AIDS or candidal blood infections, intravenous drugs like caspofungin and amphotericin B are options. These drugs themselves have serious side effects, though, and can make their users feel very sick.

More disturbingly for many patients is the fact that they have recurring symptoms or symptoms that don't seem to be "provably linked" to candida, at least for traditional medical practitioners. There has been a divide between the traditional medical community and the natural or alternative medical community for some time now concerning the existence of systemic candidiasis, a kind of hypersensitivity to candida. This is probably the very problem that has led you here, although it is not medically recognized.

You're not alone. Since Dr. William Crook published *The Yeast Connection* in 1986, the topic has been widely discussed. The general alternative medical consensus is that systemic candidiasis or candida is linked to a host of problems occurring together as a syndrome: fatigue, asthma, skin problems such as eczema and psoriasis, irritable bowel syndrome and other digestive problems, urinary tract issues, PMS, sexual dysfunction, and muscle pain or even multiple sclerosis.

The issue is that, although technically "subclinical," or too low or not localized enough to be detected by a test, candida has built up within the system of the person experiencing the symptoms, due to poor diet and possibly stress, poor health, and other factors. The idea is to eliminate excess candida with a dietary cleanse, and then to change the overall diet enough to eliminate that kind of buildup permanently.

It's easy enough to see how such a buildup might happen, given our modern American diet. Rife with convenience foods and other over-processed foods heavy with simple carbohydrates and sugars, the standard American diet is a boon to candida. Dr. Crook recommended eating a diet of fresh foods and avoiding foods high in yeast and sugars. He also postulated that fermented foods should be avoided, so no vinegars or alcohol (which is often also sugary and yeasty).

10 Signs You Might Have Candida

If you're thinking you might have candida but you're just not sure, here are 10 common signs of candida buildup in the body. If this list sounds like your own personal health complaint list, this book is definitely for you.

1. **Frequent fungal infections of the skin and nails, such as athlete's foot, toenail fungus, or skin infections under the breasts or in the armpit creases.** Fungal skin infections are sadly common for candida sufferers. That's because these kinds of infections are connected to a substandard immune system and sometimes a lack of oxygen in the blood or poor circulation. Just like other candida symptoms, these infections are signaling more serious trouble that is being caused by your weak immune system. (It is important to be cautious when checking for these skin infections, since other skin problems like eczema and psoriasis are also common in candida sufferers. These problems can look similar, so be careful, and seek medical attention whenever needed.)

2. **Feeling tired and worn down, or suffering from chronic fatigue or fibromyalgia.** Millions of Americans suffer from fatigue. Is it chronic fatigue or just feeling worn out? Research indicates that fatigue is one of the leading ailments Americans seek help for—not only conventional medical help but alternative help. Traditional medical tests often fail to explain the chronic fatigue symptoms that so many seem to experience, so this, like candida, is another ailment for which natural remedies are often sought.

   In addition to Dr. Crook, certain doctors in practice now believe that candida along with yeasts, sugars, and other foods and chemicals that can trigger sensitivities in certain people are primary causes of fatigue. These experts believe that candida and diets that foster it in the body can cause everything from simple exhaustion to headaches and even CMS.

3. **Digestive issues such as bloating, constipation, or diarrhea.** Spastic colon, irritable bowel syndrome, diarrhea (IBS), bloating, gas, and a host of digestive problems can all be related to systemic candida overload. Candida sufferers are often diagnosed with IBS and, given their irregularity, are often prescribed laxatives, especially natural

fiber treatments such as Metamucil. Since these aren't so harmful to the body even with an unsure diagnosis, they are safe for a doctor to recommend.

Unfortunately, when candida goes unrecognized, it can grow as a problem. When the candida overgrowth becomes more prolific, food ferments instead of digesting. The overgrowth can penetrate the intestinal lining, breaching the line between the intestines and the circulatory system. The entire gut becomes increasingly inflamed, and yeast is more likely to enter the bloodstream. Some people refer to this as "leaky gut," and the body's immune system starts to fight the yeast particles, leading to the next set of issues.

4. **Autoimmune diseases such as Hashimoto's thyroiditis, rheumatoid arthritis, ulcerative colitis, lupus, psoriasis, scleroderma, or multiple sclerosis.** Experts believe that food sensitivities and even allergies can develop as a result of this "leaking." This is because the yeast particles that get into the blood are fought by the immune system and then "remembered" by it the next time it sees them. This is one reason that people with candidiasis and candida overgrowth react so badly to foods containing yeast and fungi: their immune systems are primed for the bad reaction and cannot distinguish properly.

5. **Difficulty concentrating, poor memory, lack of focus, attention deficit disorder (ADD), attention deficit hyperactivity disorder (ADHD), and brain fog.** One of the most common candida-related mental complaints is brain fog or difficulty concentrating. Brain fog is a tough problem to have because, unlike a formal diagnosis of dementia, for example, there is no clear way to understand or recognize brain fog other than feeling "off," unable to concentrate, a simple lack of clarity. In other words, it is very subjective.

Recent studies have shown that ADD and ADHD and leaky gut are also linked. For this reason food allergies as well as candida are often a problem for ADD or ADHD sufferers (and vice versa). In fact, gluten and/or candida sensitivity is generally thought to precede food allergies that in turn impact ADD and ADHD. Candida overgrowth is often at the root of food allergies.

6. **Skin issues such as eczema, psoriasis, hives, and rashes.** Candida overgrowth itself causes toxins—the by-product of the yeast particles themselves—to spread throughout the body. As a result, the immune system overreacts and cannot distinguish between the candida overgrowth and other threats to the body, as discussed earlier. Psoriasis and the resulting scaly, thickened skin lesions are one such response. Unfortunately, doctors tend to prescribe anti-inflammatory and immunosuppressant drugs to fight psoriasis, and both of these can worsen candida overgrowth. Eczema presents similar issues.

7. **Irritability, mood swings, anxiety, or depression.** Among the most frightening and disturbing symptoms that candida can cause in its sufferers are the psychological symptoms. It shouldn't be surprising that the brain would be sensitive to mycotoxins, which are the toxic by-products of candida. Many experts have found that patients who are initially thought to suffer from mental or psychiatric illness are actually simply suffering from candida.

   Psychological symptoms that candida can cause include anxiety and depression. The symptoms can also present as more formal psychiatric symptoms and can include angry outbursts, irritability, mood swings, obsessive-compulsive behaviors, panic attacks, paranoia, personality changes, severe crying jags, and even behavior that might be characterized as schizophrenic. When these issues are caused by candida overgrowth and that problem is treated effectively, even these psychological symptoms dissipate without other treatment.

8. **Vaginal infections, urinary tract infections, rectal itching, or vaginal itching.** Because candida occurs naturally in the vagina, it's common for overgrowth to be apparent there. Frequent infections with or without itching are indicative of candida. Some symptoms of vaginal candidiasis include pain while urinating, itching, redness of the vulva, a thick white vaginal discharge that looks somewhat like cottage cheese, and sometimes whitish patches on the skin of the vulva. Generally discharge from this kind of infection isn't foul-smelling, although being immunocompromised can bring other kinds of infections.

   Rectal itching generally stems from candida in the vaginal or penile area. Urinary tract infections (UTIs) that are caused by candida tend to arise from candida overgrowth in the genital area. (Most UTIs, statistically, are caused by bacteria.)

9. **Severe seasonal allergies, itchy ears, or chronic sinusitis.** As already discussed, candida cells and even food particles enter your bloodstream and prompt a disproportionate immune response. This triggers inflammation and an overreaction from your immune system's specialized immune cells, called macrophages. This means that every time you eat this particular food, you end up with this same, severe immune response, and it is this hypersensitivity that gives you allergies. As you fight your allergies and the symptoms they give you, your adrenal glands work too hard and your immune system works even harder—and you have even less of what you need to fight the candida.

10. **Strong sugar and refined carbohydrate cravings.** Along with the rest of these awful symptoms, candida even makes you feel like you're fighting yourself. Yeasts ferment sugars into alcohol, and this in turn destabilizes your blood sugar level. The result? Intense and immediate cravings for even more simple carbohydrates and sugar. These organisms know how to survive.

Treatment Options Your Doctor Might Prescribe

As you begin your journey toward health, you might wonder what options your doctor would present you with. Before you get that far, how do you test for candida overgrowth?

Since many traditional medical doctors don't believe in candida overgrowth, this isn't a simple answer. However, these are some suggestions that experts recommend. Blood tests can check for high levels of IgG, IgA, and IgM candida antibodies, which can indicate candida overgrowth and can be found by a medical lab. These are less sensitive, though, than stool and urine testing, and often come back negative even when the others are positive.

Stool testing is a sensitive measure for candida, and many alternative practitioners believe it is the best way to find candida overgrowth, because it searches the colon and lower intestines for candida and can even discern the species of yeast that is causing the overgrowth. Some experts also say that stool testing can show which treatment will work for you, but these claims are only true of extended stool tests, not standard tests.

Finally, the urine organix dysbiosis test can find a candida waste product, d-arabinitol. If your result is elevated, that means you might have an overgrowth of candida, and it should also show whether it is in your upper digestive tract or your small intestine.

If your doctor determines that you are suffering from a candida overgrowth, you will face another hurdle: traditional medical treatments often exacerbate the problem.

Currently there is no truly effective treatment for CFS. As for the digestive disorders caused by candida, many sufferers are given natural fiber treatments such as Metamucil. These treatments are ineffective against the actual problem and can actually increase bloating and gas.

Furthermore, when the candida overgrowth becomes more prolific, the fermentation problem grows. The entire gut becomes increasingly inflamed, and yeast is even more likely to enter the bloodstream. Leaky gut worsens, and the body's immune system fights the yeast particles more and more, leading to more immunosuppression issues and allergies. If your issues manifest on your skin, through psoriasis or eczema for example, your doctor may prescribe anti-inflammatory and immunosuppressant drugs, which can worsen candida overgrowth.

In the end, you may find that conventional medical treatment worsens your mental symptoms. These cycles of ineffective treatment and deteriorating health can be frustrating and depressing.

2

CANDIDA AND FOOD

As they say, you are what you eat, and when it comes to candida that is definitely true. Although the symptoms of candida can feel overwhelming, the fact that candida overgrowth and diet are so interconnected means that you can take control of your symptoms. But first, here's how it works.

How Does Diet Affect Candida?

Typically, the healthy bacteria in your body keep your candida levels in balance. However, there are many factors—especially in modern American life—that can cause the candida population to grow out of control.

Eating a diet high in sugar and simple, processed, or refined carbohydrates causes candida to grow out of control and blood sugar levels to vary dramatically. The result is a vicious cycle that perpetuates itself.

Blood glucose comes from foods or other nutrients in the body, including from glucose already stored in the muscles. When your blood sugar gets low, your body either makes more or uses up stored sugar.

If your blood sugar gets high, your body secretes insulin until your blood sugar is back in the good range.

Sugars and simple carbohydrates are food for yeast, pure and simple. The conditions in your belly are perfect for fermenting both sugar and yeast into alcohol. This fermentation is part of the metabolic process in which your body converts carbohydrates like starches and sugars into alcohols to obtain energy. Obviously your body needs energy, and this is a positive process. However, modern American diets tend to be far too high in sugars and processed carbohydrates, leading to cyclic, intense cravings for even more simple carbohydrates and sugar.

As you feel these cravings, you already know what happens: Sooner or later, you give in. This is especially true when your lifestyle is busy and stressful and you find yourself rushing. At the last minute you end up feeling starved, and these cravings feel strong. This leads you to be far more likely to choose more sugary, simple carbohydrates and highly processed foods.

It goes without saying that this is a gold mine for many American food producers. It's no secret that this kind of eating cycle is habit-forming. The part that has remained hidden for many is its effects on their overall health.

You already know that eating this way can make you fat, and you know that you can have a vague feeling that you're just "run down" or "not feeling so hot." But the idea that you may have serious, chronic health problems as a result of a white-bread and high-sugar diet really is difficult for many people to accept, especially in a culture that has traditionally equated happiness with things like cake, ice cream, burgers, and fries.

The Candida Cleanse and Diet

If you suffer from candida overgrowth symptoms, you can take charge of the problem once and for all. The pain and discomfort you are feeling justifies at least trying to do that.

You might have seen a medical doctor about the problem, but it didn't work. It's been enough of a problem for you that you've decided to research the issue on your own. The real question is, what do you have to lose by simply changing the foods you eat for a set period of time, in the name of your health—and why would you resist doing that when you might find that the diet change was all it took?

There are two basic steps in the candida cleanse and diet. First you cleanse, and then you transition into the diet. You transition only once your body is ready and your health has improved enough to justify that step, but generally speaking you will cleanse only for 14 days. Isn't that worth trying?

This isn't to say it's easy. It takes effort. Just like quitting smoking or losing weight, changing the way you look at sugar, yeast, and carbohydrates takes work. Furthermore, depending on how serious your problem with candida is, you might need a multipronged approach. Using diet alone to control candida overgrowth can take three to six months, and this is assuming that you do not have a more serious problem such as clinical candidiasis.

Because of this many people do seek the assistance of a doctor while they cleanse, and some also use antifungal medications such as fluconazole or nystatin as they change their diets (as appropriate, of course). If your condition does not merit this kind of drug, you can try a caprylic acid supplement. Caprylic acid is derived from coconut oil and is also found naturally in palm oil and both human and cow's milk. It has been found by the U.S. Food and Drug Administration (FDA) to be generally safe, although it has not been approved yet for what it is most commonly used for: killing yeast.

Oil of oregano is also commonly used to kill yeast by those who are treating candida overgrowth; however, it is also harmful to some varieties of beneficial bacteria. Since candida overgrowth itself is a massive systemic imbalance, use of oil of oregano is not recommended here. Instead, stick to those treatments that are specific to yeast, including whatever prescription antifungals your doctor deems necessary for your health, and supplements such as caprylic acid and probiotics.

In the cleansing stage, you will strip all yeasts, sugars, breads, simple carbohydrates, grains, fruits, most dairy, many vegetables, and almost all processed foods from your diet.

Sounds intimidating, doesn't it? You will find, using the tips and recipes in this cookbook, that you can do it. You will also find that the way you feel is far better than you expected. In fact, your body is going to feel so different, you may not believe it.

In fairly short order, you will transition into the next stage, which is far easier. You will add more vegetables back into your routine, along with some fruits. You'll find yourself feeling like more of an "old pro" with the regimen, and you may even see yourself losing weight as an unintended fringe benefit of the diet. (Please see the note below if you are someone who needs to maintain or gain weight while cleansing your body of candida overgrowth.)

Does it sound too good to be true? Remember, it isn't easy. Sugars and yeasts really are addictive. Yeast is a survivor. You will find yourself feeling intense cravings. Use the tools in this book to fight them and take back your health.

One of the main (and temporary) side effects of a candida cleanse is the Jarisch-Herxheimer reaction, named after the Austrian dermatologist Adolf Jarisch and the German dermatologist Karl Herxheimer. This refers to how, for a day or two, your symptoms may appear to worsen before they get better. They aren't getting worse. This reaction happens because when a large number of harmful bacteria die off in your body, naturally they release toxins. As a result, you might experience chills, fatigue, fever, headache, muscle pain, and skin breakouts. On the other hand, you might not have any of these effects at all.

Criticism of the Candida Cleanse and Diet

There are many experts and medical doctors who do not subscribe to the idea that candida overgrowth is an actual health problem. There are also some more common-sense criticisms. In the interest of giving you all the facts, that perspective is detailed here so you may judge for yourself.

The American Academy of Allergy, Asthma, and Immunology (AAAAI) has released a position statement saying that the idea of a hypersensitivity to candida is unproven. The statement expresses concern that this is problematic not only because the elements of the syndrome are very broad and could apply to almost anyone, but also because it may be causing well people to be overusing antifungal drugs. This in turn might lead to the creation of drug resistance and possible side effects, although these are reportedly very rare. There have been no controlled trials to study these issues. Allergic symptoms in particular are influenced by a host of factors, including mental ones (as are most symptoms).

It is illegal in the United States for any person or entity to sell any product to prevent or treat a disease without FDA approval. Anything sold for those purposes is considered to be a "drug," even if the seller doesn't call it that. Back in the 1980s, Nature's Way sold "natural supplements" that were slated to cure yeast infections—not candida overgrowth, but actual yeast infections. In 1989, the FDA's fraud branch caught up with this practice and in 1990 Nature's Way stopped selling this product, and paid a $30,000 settlement to the National Institutes of Health as a part of their agreement based on their admission of wrongdoing.

Also in 1990, two New Jersey doctors were barred from diagnosing candida overgrowth syndrome, as it had not yet been generally recognized.

A commonsense criticism of the cleanse and diet stems from the fact that they are highly restrictive. Especially in the cleansing stage, many very nutritious foods are eliminated, and the consumption of carbohydrates is severely limited. This means that many of the symptoms relating to fatigue, mood swings, depression, poor concentration, and brain fog might be exacerbated.

The Mayo Clinic is skeptical about the candida cleanse's ability to cure candida, although they acknowledge its health benefits in general. Since most people who take up the cleanse and diet cut sugar and white flour out of their diet, as a result they eliminate most processed foods. This means that by following the candida cleanse and diet, they cut out foods that are higher in calories and lower in nutritional value. The bottom line for the Mayo Clinic? After you do that for enough time, you will eventually feel better, have more energy, and improve your health overall. That is the benefit of the cleanse and diet, in their eyes.

Addressing these criticisms one by one, the AAAAI position statement is certainly notable. There is no question that the syndrome itself is not proven and that there have been no clinical trials. Also, there is never a justification for using a prescription drug without cause; this is why you must be sure to be under the care of a medical doctor for that portion of your treatment. However, without clinical trials, what remains is anecdotal evidence, and there is simply no question that many, many people have been helped by the candida cleanse and diet after nothing else worked. Given that the primary complaint of the AAAAI focuses on the prescription drug issue, there is little reason to eschew the cleanse and diet based on the position statement.

The Nature's Way case and isolated New Jersey doctor incidents in 1990 are certainly worth considering. However, the vitamin supplement itself is a specific case of one product, and one that was geared toward curing an actual vaginal yeast infection. It isn't clear what was in the supplement, but the cleanse and diet are more akin to a lifestyle change. Furthermore, the actions of a business are, by necessity, treated with far more scrutiny than should be the decisions made by individual people as they choose what to eat.

Taking up the issue of the restrictiveness of the cleanse and diet, this is something very important to consider. Anytime you follow a more restrictive regimen, it is absolutely crucial to monitor your body's response closely, not just for the symptoms mentioned previously, but for any negative responses. If you experience major difficulty adjusting, you should change your approach. Every body is different, and each person's caloric needs are unique. As you need to adjust your intake, you will.

Given that this cleanse and diet allows for three meals, two snacks, and one dessert each day, it is unlikely that you will be hungry if you follow it. And if you find yourself hungry, eat more from your list. Finally, if your health fails in any way, you should discontinue your cleanse.

As the Mayo Clinic concluded, when you change your diet and make healthy changes, you are likely to be in better health. There is really no reason to refuse to try this cleanse and diet, if you are suffering from candida overgrowth symptoms. If you are likely to feel better anyway, you have no excuses left.

3

EATING WITH CANDIDA

You might be thinking by now that this diet is too hard, that you can't stick with it. Well, think again. First, consider these 10 easy rules for relieving candida symptoms through your diet and habits. Even when you can't get to your guidelines and you're unsure about details, these simple rules of thumb will help keep you centered and on track (and your candida under control).

10 Tips for Relieving the Symptoms of Candida Through Your Diet

1. **If it's sweet, do not eat.** You already know that all sugars, even natural ones that occur in fruit, feed candida. You also know that all artificial sweeteners are off the list and that stevia is your only ally here. Just remember that foods that are sweet are always sweetened by something, and chances are excellent that whatever that source of sweetness is feeds candida. Don't eat it.

    On the other hand, do always try to keep packets of stevia on hand, at work, in your bag, and at the gym. This way if you decide to have some herbal tea while you're out, you can have some sweetness while you're at it.

2.   **Bitter is better.** Bitter foods such as aloe vera juice (in its pure state), dandelion greens and roots, endive, jicama, mustard greens, radicchio, radishes, spinach, and other leafy greens counteract cravings for sweets. (Lemon juice does, too.) They contain enzymes that aid digestion and improve kidney and liver function. If you counteract sweet cravings with bitter foods, you will slowly combat them.

3.   **Start totaling the tees.** All alcohol is food for candida overgrowth and must be eliminated. Furthermore, consider the damaging properties of alcohol generally, as discussed below.

4.   **Water, water, water.** As with any flush of the system, with this diet you cannot get too much water. Your system needs it right now, for so many reasons. You are trying to eliminate toxins from your body and cleanse your renal system. Dehydration is an ongoing health issue for most of us. There is very little downside to drinking water.

5.   **Avoid even beneficial fermented foods like kombucha, sauerkraut, and pickles, except apple cider vinegar, kefir, and probiotic yogurt.** Because fermentation in the gut and resultant leaking is such a problem with candida overgrowth, it is best to avoid even healthful fermented foods during your cleanse, except as noted.

6.   **Address your stress.** This is the one tip that is not strictly diet related, but it is so important and connected to the entire problem (as well as the cleanse) that it belongs here anyway. There is no question that excessive stress is at the heart of many human illnesses, and candida overgrowth is one of the most seriously impacted by stress. Just as your appetite is affected by your stress levels, so is the rest of the problem.

7.   **Take antibiotics and oral contraceptives sparingly and carefully, and consume probiotics like a pro.** Always take a good probiotic supplement, in either capsule or powder form, especially if you have to take antibiotics or oral contraceptives. These come packing anything from 1 billion to 100 billion or more bacteria per dose, and typically it is best to start conservatively and then increase the dosage. Some supplements contain only one kind of bacteria, and others contain more than a dozen. As long as the most effective strains are present, the probiotic will work well. *Lactobacillus acidophilus* or *Bifidobacterium bifidum* are the most common and are also very effective. *L. acidophilus* DDS-1, a more potent strain, is even better. Some probiotics contain prebiotics, which are supposed to help the probiotics work, but these are not needed.

8.   **Make it from scratch whenever you can.** When you make it yourself, you know exactly what's in it. Try to prepare everything you can yourself and you'll eliminate the guesswork about what you're eating.

9.   **When eating out, keep it simple.** Fancy sauces, preparations, and sides are almost always danger areas for the candida cleanse. You need to be able to identify everything on your plate and ensure it isn't prepared with anything that's off your list.

10. **When it doubt, leave it out.** It can be so tempting to take a chance, but don't. If you're not 100 percent sure about something being on your safe list, don't eat it. After a while, you'll be so glad you followed this policy, because once you experience the feeling of candida being cleared and then have a relapse, the rush of symptoms returning will feel much worse than they did before.

Foods to Avoid

Additives and preservatives: citric acid and anything you can't identify or pronounce. The additive form of citric acid that is manufactured is yeast-based, although the natural form, which is found in lemons and limes, is fine. Any other additives and preservatives can disrupt healthy bacteria and cause an imbalance.

Alcohol: beer, cider, liquor, spirits, wine. Alcohol is high in sugars and, therefore, instant food for candida. It's also hard on your body and your immune system. Once alcohol is in your system, it is metabolized first, because it cannot be stored in the body, unlike protein, carbohydrates, and fat. As you recall, sugars are broken down into alcohol; consumed alcohol is already broken down. Once alcohol enters your stomach, up to 20 percent of it is absorbed there and enters your bloodstream directly. In other words, it acts like instant sugar and usurps all other more nutritional energy sources.

Avoid it no matter what.

Artificial sweeteners except stevia. Even sweeteners like aspartame in diet soda and tea weaken your immune system.

Beans and legumes: beans, chickpeas, legumes, all soy products, including tofu. Although they are healthful, because these foods are tough to digest and relatively high in carbohydrates, they cannot be eaten during the initial cleanse portion of the diet. Bring them back later in small amounts. Unfortunately, all soy products are off the list, as the majority of soy products are genetically modified (GMO).

Beverages with caffeine or that are decaffeinated (they once had caffeine): coffee, black and green tea, soda, diet soda, energy drinks. Caffeine forces your blood sugar to jump or "spike," which puts a burden on your immune system. Coffee and some kinds of tea also contain mold. Even teas and coffees that have been decaffeinated contain some caffeine.

Condiments: ketchup, horseradish, mayonnaise (except when you make it yourself using the recipe in this book), regular yellow mustard, relish, salad dressings (except the ones you make from the recipes in this book), soy sauce, tomato paste, tomato sauce. All of these contain high amounts of hidden sugars. For an alternative salad dressing, try a simple olive oil and lemon juice dressing. Dry mustard from your spice rack is okay, too.

Dairy products: buttermilk, cheese, cream, ice cream, milk. Almost all dairy should be avoided except butter, ghee, kefir, and probiotic yogurt. Milk and anything else containing lactose must be avoided because lactose is a kind of sugar. Kefir and yogurt are better choices; almost all the lactose disappears as they ferment.

Fats and oils: canola oil, corn oil, peanut oil, soy oil. Baked goods made with canola oil, corn oil, and peanut oil develop mold very quickly. Most soybeans used in soy oil are GMO (genetically modified organisms).

Fish: all fish and shellfish except anchovies, herring, wild salmon, and sardines. All shellfish and most fish are far too high in heavy metals and toxins, which suppress the immune system. Farmed salmon contains high levels of PCBs (polychlorinated biphenyls), mercury, and other carcinogens.

Fruit: any fruit—canned, dried, fresh, or juiced. An occasional spritz of lemon juice as a dressing is okay. Fruit is too high in natural sugars to be eaten while eliminating candida, although some fresh fruit can be introduced later. Dried fruit in particular has a very high sugar content and must be avoided, and this is also true of fruit juice and canned fruit. Some melons such as cantaloupe also have moldy rinds, and discarding the rind does not mean avoiding the mold altogether.

Fungi: mushrooms and truffles. Some mushrooms and fungi are harmful if you are already suffering from candida, but some mushrooms are good in the diet, including maitake and reishi.

Grains, gluten: barley, bread of any kind, corn, corn products, oats, pasta, rice, rice products, rye, spelt, wheat, wheat products. Candida overgrowth and gluten sensitivity go hand in hand, and many grains, especially popcorn, are contaminated with mold. All yeast bread is off limits, thanks to the yeast.

Meats: pork and any pork products, any meat that is canned, cured, processed, smoked, or vacuum-packed, lunch meats. Pork is dangerous for those with digestive problems because it contains bacteria that survive cooking. Processed meats such as lunch meat contain additives like dextrose, nitrates, and sulfates, not to mention sugars.

Nuts: cashews, peanuts, pistachios. These kinds of nuts are very susceptible to mold.

Sugars: brown sugar, granulated sugar, honey, maple syrup, molasses, powdered sugar, rice syrup. Condiments and dressings are filled with sugar. Always read labels. Assume restaurant food is far more sugary than you think.

Vegetables: beets, carrots, parsnips, peas, potatoes, sweet potatoes, yams. These are very healthful foods, but they can only be reintroduced one at a time once your cleanse is over and your overgrowth is under control.

Vinegar: any variety except unfiltered apple cider vinegar. Because vinegars are made using yeast cultures and can cause inflammation in your gut, they have to be avoided. This is true of all vinegars except unfiltered apple cider vinegar.

Foods to Enjoy

Beverages and brews: chicory root coffee; tea made from cinnamon, ginger, licorice, or peppermint; water; freshly juiced vegetables on your safe list. These brewed drinks are all antifungal, and chicory root can also help your gut rebalance itself with healthy flora. When juicing vegetables, aim in particular for leafy greens, which counteract cravings for sweets. They also contain enzymes that aid with digestion and improve kidney and liver function.

Eggs, including mayonnaise you make yourself with the recipe in this book. Look for fresh organic eggs. Cook eggs in fats that are on your list.

Fish: anchovies, herring, sardines, wild salmon. These varieties of fish (and no others) have acceptable levels of contaminants for candida sufferers. Choose only fresh or those packed in water or olive oil.

Fruits: avocados, unsweetened cranberries, unsweetened rhubarb, lemons, limes. After your cleanse and the elimination of your symptoms, you may reintroduce apples, blueberries, peaches, pears, pineapples, raspberries, and strawberries in small amounts.

Grains: buckwheat, millet, oat bran, quinoa. These high-fiber foods help your digestive tract move well and get rid of candida waste products. You can also feel free to use products from these grains, like buckwheat flour.

Herbs and spices: basil, black pepper, cinnamon, cloves, dill, garlic, ginger, oregano, paprika, rosemary, thyme. Herbs and spices are natural antifungal agents and many can also act as anti-inflammatories. They are also your best friends when you are on a limited diet.

Live yogurt cultures: kefir, probiotic yogurt. Live cultures in yogurt help your body fight overgrowth of candida and repopulate your gut with healthy bacteria. The living cultures in the yogurt bring the bacterial balance back to your system. Always try this after taking antibiotics.

Meats: beef, chicken, lamb, turkey. Eat only fresh meats and never any processed, packed, smoked, vacuum-packed, or lunch meats. Choose organic meats whenever possible.

Nuts and seeds: almonds, coconut, flax seeds, hazelnuts, pecans, sunflower seeds, walnuts. These nuts and seeds are great for you and have a low enough mold content for you to safely enjoy.

Oils and fats: almond oil, butter, coconut oil, flax oil, ghee, lard, macadamia oil, mayonnaise you make with the recipe in this book, olive oil, red palm oil, sesame oil, sunflower oil, coconut oil, walnut oil. These oils are all safe and healthful for you to use. Whenever you can, use cold-pressed oils, as this process preserves the oil's nutrients. Olive oil and coconut oil are best for cooking, and coconut oil is best at high heat. Extra-virgin olive oil can smoke at high temperatures. Many seed oils, including flax seed oil, sunflower oil, and sesame oil, are not good for cooking.

Seasonings (other than spices): apple cider vinegar, black pepper, coconut aminos, lemon juice, sea salt. Try making dressings with olive oil, either apple cider vinegar or lemon juice, and salt and pepper. You'll find coconut aminos a fantastic alternative to soy sauce when you want something different.

Sweetener: stevia. This is your one totally safe bet for candida.

Vegetables: artichokes, asparagus, bok choy, broccoli, broccoli rabe, Brussels sprouts, cabbage, carrots, cauliflower, celery, chard, cucumber, eggplant, garlic, kale, leeks, olives, onions, rutabaga, shallots, spinach, tomatoes, zucchini. Non-starchy vegetables are perfect for your cleanse. They help you starve the candida. You should always buy your vegetables as fresh as you can, and organic whenever possible. Eat them grilled, steamed, or best of all, raw. Avoid starchy vegetables (as you've already seen from the earlier list). Olives are an acceptable treat as long as they are not prepared in vinegar.

Additional Help

Use antimicrobial and antifungal herbs and foods. Agrimony, andrographis, barberry, bitter orange, black cumin, black walnut, cloves, dandelion, echinacea, garlic, gentian, golden seal, neem, olive leaf, onions, Oregon grape, pau d'arco, rhubarb, thyme, and wormwood are antiparasitic and anti-infective, and protect the liver. Include them in your diet fresh or in good-quality supplements without additives.

Restore the healthy balance of normal bacterial flora in your body. Take *L. acidophilus* and bifidobacteria *B. bifidus* supplements every day. These supplements also reduce symptoms such as bloating, constipation, thrush, and yeast infections.

Repair the integrity of your gastrointestinal membranes. Eat glutamine-rich foods such as Brussels sprouts, celery, dandelion greens, lettuce, parsley, and spinach.

Shopping Tips

Now that you have a sense of what to look for, shopping for yourself is crucial. This is because so much of the food that you buy in restaurants or already prepared in a store is off limits. Even prepared food that sounds or looks healthful can be deceiving, so it's important to have a supply of fresh "safety" food at home. That way, sticking to your new goals is much easier.

You don't have to be a cook to do this, but you still need to shop. Here are some easy tips to help you make your kitchen a strong anti-candida front line.

Shop for small amounts of fresh food frequently. Even though it can be tempting to tick various items off your shopping list—particularly when they are specialty items, as they often are during a candida cleanse—resist the urge to over-shop. Of course, if you need basics that last on a shelf, you can stock up. However, even grains and jarred items should be as fresh as you can get them. Especially when you're trying to beat candida, you need to choose the fresh option instead of any other whenever possible.

When you get into the habit of small, frequent trips, you will find yourself more likely to shop according to your cleanse rules, too. A daily or every-other-day stroll by a fresh meat or fish counter and produce stand will let you choose what looks best and appeals to you right now. It also helps you avoid waste.

Frequent stores that are a reliable source for organic foods. Not only will this habit let you access organic choices, but you are also more likely to find unusual and alternative food choices that candida sufferers seek out.

Become a habitual label reader. This is probably the most important tip. Never assume you know what's in something just because you know what it is, even when you've had it a million times, and even when you're certain it's something that's very good for your health. Once you start down this road and commit to eliminating your candida overgrowth, you have to be certain you are eradicating all sources of it from reentering your body.

If there is anything on the label that you're unsure of, put it down. Anything you can't pronounce? Put it down. Even a very small amount of something you shouldn't have? Put it down. You will find yourself putting down almost everything in bottles, jars, and boxes, and that's good.

Dining Out

Just as with any cleanse or new food regime, eating out can be challenging at first. It's not impossible, though, and with a few habits to keep in mind, you can do it whenever you want or need to.

Don't see dining out as a splurge. Although it's easy to see eating out as a special occasion (and sometimes it is), don't get into that mind-set when you choose what you'll eat. That just makes it easier to stray from your acceptable foods list. Instead, try to see eating out as being in someone else's house, or otherwise being a traveler in need of safe foods. Keep a "safe and frugal" mind-set as you consider your choices.

Ask lots of questions. Not all food servers are thrilled to play Twenty Questions with you about the menu, but that's their job, especially these days, when people have special needs, from allergies to diabetes. Speak up. Here are some examples.

If you're going to order grilled salmon, make sure it's wild-caught. You also need to know what they put on it before it's grilled. There is virtually no chance that it doesn't have some kind of preparation on it, and any kind of marinade feeds your candida. However, there is also just about a 100 percent certainty that the chef also has olive oil, and if they just brush it with olive oil, grill it, and bring it to you with a lemon wedge, you're in the clear.

Bring your own supplies if you need to. As mentioned earlier, you should bring things like stevia with you, and if there are other supplies that you find key to your success, bring them. If you are sure you're going to need coconut aminos at a Chinese restaurant and you know they won't have them, bring them.

Take advantage of accommodations for allergies and similar situations. Everyone is much more aware of food allergies these days, and restaurateurs more so than most. Treat your cleanse diet as if you are simply dealing with a host of food allergies; after all, you are avoiding foods that have made you seriously ill over time. Talk to your server and, if necessary, the chef, about your "allergies," and take advantage of their skill and creativity. You may be pleasantly surprised at what they come up with; after all, they genuinely do want you to enjoy your meal and will often endeavor to make that happen.

When you can choose where to eat, make sure it's a good option. When your friend calls and asks if you'd rather hit The Bread Factory or Natural Green Kitchen, choose the one that makes the most sense for your cleanse. And if that difference isn't apparent or you're not familiar with any of the options, take a few minutes and check them out. It'll save you trouble and frustration later. If you eat out for business frequently, you can have a "safe" list for when it's your turn to choose, and you can get comfortable with what safe choices you have at different restaurants.

Maintaining Health After Candida

One of the best ways to maintain your health after restoring it is to see yourself on the cusp of a new lifestyle. Someone who has given up a dangerous addiction in favor of health foods and exercise isn't seen as switching to a lifestyle of deprivation, and neither are you.

Have you ever been to a yoga class where the people were living raw-food, candida-free, macrobiotic, or similar lifestyles? If so, you were in a group where even in your post-candida reality you would feel as if you were in the majority. This is the kind of situation you may need to experience from time to time, to remind yourself that it's not deprivation or denial, but the positive gift of health and physical ability that is your focus.

Here are some tips for maintaining your health once you've transitioned away from cleansing.

Remember what it was like being sick. Not that you want to dwell on the bad things in life, but never forget why you're doing what you're doing. And once you're through it all and you've regained your health, never forget how sick you really were at times. It is the natural way of the human body and its amazing knack for survival to blur painful memories, and memories about pain you've suffered will indeed become cloudy. That's a good thing.

However, as you begin you might want to record your thoughts as you experience your symptoms. Write down how you feel on a particularly miserable night. Take a picture of your poor, swollen belly when it's hurting. Do something to remind yourself of how bad your symptoms really are when you don't take care of them. It can help you strengthen your resolve in times of good health.

Celebrate being healthy. On the positive side, celebrate your health success. Think of all of the things you can do now that used to be impossible. One woman pointed out that she could sit comfortably for hours with friends and not be annoyed by itching skin. Another mentioned that she could play bridge again, without brain fog making it impossible. One man said that without terrible fatigue he was able to run again.

Whatever you can do now or do again, celebrate it. Photograph it, tell your friends, make it a big deal.

Take up a new hobby or activity that you couldn't have done when you weren't as healthy. Did you ever wish to try something like yoga but didn't feel you could? Have your digestive issues in the past made you embarrassed in social situations? Now that you're learning a candida-free lifestyle, celebrate your good health by taking up something new that you wouldn't have in the past.

You used to simply live with your symptoms, and before you knew it you changed your life in so many ways, large and small. Now, change it again.

Find friends and acquaintances who have made similar lifestyle changes, for mutual support. Another great way to keep your fire burning is to stoke it with friends. You may think candida overgrowth is too obscure, but you're probably wrong. It's actually very common.

Still, you don't need to find friends who have done the very same thing to get the support you need. Millions of people every day decide to quit smoking, quit drinking alcohol, eliminate gluten from their diets, whatever it is that is causing their health to suffer. When you talk to people who have been through a similar journey, you will find that there is strength in numbers.

Stay creative. Finally, even once you've gotten the hang of things and settled into your new lifestyle, a routine doesn't have to mean a rut. Be creative. Look for new recipes in places like this book and online, and share with your friends. The more the merrier, and your own imagination may prove you to be an innovator.

4

14-DAY CLEANSE MEAL PROGRAM

Now to the business of your meal program and how it works. This chapter shows you in a 14-day stretch exactly how your cleanse breaks down. From Day 1 through Day 14, each day will include a breakfast, midmorning snack, lunch, midday snack, dinner, and dessert. You can keep yourself both healthy and satisfied. Each of these 14 sample days includes at least one recipe from this book (denoted with a *) so you can see how it all fits together.

Day 1

Breakfast: Grown-up Green Eggs*
Midmorning Snack: Veggie sticks and dip
Lunch: Chicken "Noodle" Soup*
Midday Snack: Jicama Fries*
Dinner: Roasted salmon with green salad
Dessert: Yogurt with stevia

Day 2

Breakfast: Steak and eggs
Midmorning Snack: Buckwheat muffin
Lunch: Turkey Zucchini Burger*
Midday Snack: Guacamole* and Corn-Free Chips*
Dinner: Grilled chicken and vegetables
Dessert: No-Bake Coconut Chews*

Day 3

Breakfast: Quinoa Hot Cereal*
Midmorning Snack: Almonds and hazelnuts
Lunch: Grilled salmon salad
Midday Snack: Broccoli and dip
Dinner: Coconut Fried Chicken* and Mashed Notatoes*
Dessert: Almond muffin

Day 4

Breakfast: Egg salad
Midmorning Snack: Quinoa Crackers* and Yogurt Cheese*
Lunch: Almond-butter sandwich
Midday Snack: Cold roasted asparagus and peppers
Dinner: Coconut Chicken with Spinach*
Dessert: Lemon Pudding*

Day 5

Breakfast: Breakfast sandwich
Midmorning Snack: Granola
Lunch: Beef and Okra Stew*
Midday Snack: Crackers and dip
Dinner: Herbed Salmon*
Dessert: Custard

Day 6

Breakfast: Yogurt and granola
Midmorning Snack: Deviled Eggs*
Lunch: Soup and salad
Midday Snack: Grilled Fennel Dippers*
Dinner: Coconut Lamb Curry*
Dessert: Truffles

Day 7

Breakfast: Eggs and leftover chicken
Midmorning Snack: Bread and butter
Lunch: Macadamia Nut "Hummus"* with Onion Herb Crackers*
Midday Snack: Pâté and veggies
Dinner: Steak with Ginger Sauce*
Dessert: Green Machine Smoothie*

Day 8

Breakfast: Grain-Free Pancakes* with Butter and Sweet Almond Sauce*
Midmorning Snack: Celery and Ranch Dressing*
Lunch: Sandwich
Midday Snack: Yogurt
Dinner: Soup and salad
Dessert: Coconut Chocolate Brittle*

Day 9

Breakfast: Muffin
Midmorning Snack: Crudités
Lunch: Gazpacho* and Lemony Kale Chips*
Midday Snack: Radishes and dip
Dinner: Grilled Lime Chicken Sandwich* and No-Potato Salad*
Dessert: No-bake cookies

Day 10

Breakfast: Potato-Free Hash Browns*
Midmorning Snack: Toasted onions
Lunch: Cucumbers and Tzatziki*
Midday Snack: Soup
Dinner: Tandoori Lamb*
Dessert: Nutty Seedy Truffles*

Day 11

Breakfast: Porridge the Candida-Safe Way*
Midmorning Snack: Chips and dip
Lunch: Chicken and salad
Midday Snack: Jicama and dip
Dinner: Cabbage Rolls*
Dessert: Yogurt Pudding*

Day 12

Breakfast: Fried Eggs with Grilled Avocado and Coconut Bread*
Midmorning Snack: Celery and nut butter
Lunch: Soup and crackers
Midday Snack: Buckwheat Tortillas* with Yogurt Cheese*
Dinner: Spinach and herring salad
Dessert: Carob Clusters*

Day 13

Breakfast: Grain-Free Pancakes* and eggs
Midmorning Snack: Kasha
Lunch: Quinoa Tabbouleh*
Midday Snack: Bell pepper strips and dip
Dinner: Lamb Pasticcio*
Dessert: Coconut and yogurt with stevia

Day 14

Breakfast: Eggs and toast
Midmorning Snack: Yogurt
Lunch: Roasted vegetables
Midday Snack: Sardine Pâté* and crackers
Dinner: Sautéed Wilted Kale Salad* and Broccoli Soup*
Dessert: Carob Fudge*

PART 2

Recipes to Help Eliminate Candida

5

BREAKFAST (CLEANSE)

B reakfast is the most important meal of the day, and even more so for those going through the candida cleanse. This is your opportunity to signal to your body that it is not going to be hungry all day—not to mention your chance for a delicious start to the morning.

In this chapter:

Quinoa Hot Cereal

Potato-Free Hash Browns

Coconut Muffins

Grown-Up Green Eggs

Porridge the
　　Candida-Safe Way

Grain-Free Pancakes

Simple Veggie Omelet

Buckwheat Hot Cereal

Coconut Granola Parfait

Avocado Omelet

Eggs and Turkey Not-Sausage

Breakfast Sandwich

Rhubarb Yogurt Parfait

Quinoa Hot Cereal

Makes 4 Servings

Hot, hearty grain cereals stick with you long after the old, cold cereals you used to eat did. And they have none of the sugary bad guys you're avoiding.

- 2 cups coconut milk or almond milk (plus more for serving)
- 1 cup rinsed quinoa
- Stevia to taste
- Ground cinnamon to taste
- Unsweetened cranberries and/or coconut, if desired

1. Bring milk to a boil in a small saucepan. Add quinoa and return to a boil. Reduce heat to low and simmer, covered, until around three-fourths of the milk has been absorbed, about 15 minutes.

2. Stir in stevia and cinnamon. Cook, covered, until almost all the milk has been absorbed, about 8 minutes. (You'll know the consistency you like for the cereal when you see it; feel free to cook more or less, or add more or less milk until it's just how you like it.)

3. Stir in cranberries and/or coconut and cook for 30 seconds. Serve with additional coconut or almond milk, stevia, cinnamon, cranberries, and coconut.

Potato-Free Hash Browns

Makes 2 Servings

Take advantage of how healthful (and delicious!) jicama is with this recipe. You can also add leftover meat to dress it up.

- 1 tablespoon coconut oil
- 1 small yellow onion, diced
- 4 ounces cooked meat of your choice, diced
- 2 cloves garlic, minced
- 2 cups cubed jicama
- Breakfast seasoning (recipe on page 216)
- 3 tablespoons water

---

1. Add coconut oil and diced onions to a large frying pan. Cook on medium-high heat for 5 minutes, stirring frequently.

2. Add diced meat and garlic and cook for 3 minutes, continuing to stir. Drop in cubed jicama and seasoning. Cook for a total of 10 minutes, adding 1 tablespoon water every couple of minutes and stirring to avoid burning. If you wish, serve with eggs, sunny-side up.

Coconut Muffins

Makes 6 Muffins

If you know you'll be on the run, keep these candida-safe muffins on hand. Some of the varieties in this book are extra eggy and hearty, but these are light and sweet. Take advantage of the variety.

- 2 tablespoons coconut oil, melted into liquid form, plus more for greasing muffin tin
- 3 eggs
- Coconut milk and liquid stevia to make up ¼ cup total
- ¼ teaspoon sea salt
- ¼ cup sifted coconut flour
- ¼ teaspoon baking powder
- 3 tablespoons shredded, unsweetened coconut

---

1. Preheat oven to 400°F. Grease a 6-muffin tin with coconut oil or use paper muffin cups. Set aside.

2. In a small bowl beat eggs, coconut oil, milk and stevia mixture, and salt. Combine coconut flour and baking powder, and whisk into batter until smooth.

3. Fill muffin cups half full with batter and sprinkle with shredded coconut. Bake in preheated oven for 15 to 20 minutes.

Grown-up Green Eggs

Makes 1 Serving

Even if you are Sam-I-Am, you will definitely love these. With the power of serious protein from eggs and antioxidants from kale, this is a serious breakfast that will keep you going all day, with just a few ingredients.

- 2 large kale leaves, raw, untrimmed, with stems
- 2 eggs
- Sea salt to taste
- Oil of your choice for skillet

1. Use a food processor or blender to turn your kale leaves into a purée.

2. Beat eggs. Combine eggs and kale purée and add salt. Scramble eggs in an oiled, nonstick skillet over medium-high heat. Serve with a clean, candida-safe meat—not ham.

Porridge the Candida-Safe Way

Makes 3–4 Servings

It may sound old-fashioned, but porridge is actually warm, delicious, and satisfying. It also gives you a lot of freedom because you can use whatever add-ins you love.

- 4 tablespoons chopped fresh coconut meat
- 1 tablespoon each pumpkin seeds, flax seeds, and chia seeds
- ¼ cup walnuts
- ¼ cup pecans
- 1 teaspoon ground cinnamon
- ½ teaspoon ground ginger
- 2 cups boiling milk of your choice (you may substitute water, or use half milk and half water)
- ¼ teaspoon sea salt or to taste
- Stevia, if desired
- Nuts, seeds, shredded coconut, or other extras for garnish

1. Use a food processor or blender to combine the first six ingredients except milk and/or water at a high enough speed to grind everything very finely.

2. Add milk (or water) and mix on lowest setting. Increase speed one setting at a time until you reach the highest and your porridge is smooth.

3. Heat if preferred. Serve sweetened with stevia as desired. Garnish as desired.

Grain-Free Pancakes

Makes 3–4 Servings of 2 Pancakes Each

You may have thought that giving up grain meant giving up treats like pancakes, but think again.

- 2/3 cup candida-safe flour (in the maintenance stage, use chickpea flour)
- 1 teaspoon ground cinnamon
- 1 teaspoon baking powder
- 1/2 to 2/3 cup milk of your choice
- Oil of your choice for pan
- 3 eggs
- 1 teaspoon vanilla extract

1. Combine flour, cinnamon, and baking powder in a medium-sized bowl and stir just enough to break up the bigger lumps.

2. Add milk, eggs, and vanilla and combine.

3. Heat a nonstick pan and lightly oil. Cook pancakes over medium heat until bubbles form, about 2 minutes. Reduce heat slightly and turn pancakes. Cook 2 to 3 minutes more or until done.

Simple Veggie Omelet

Makes 1 Serving

You can't go wrong eating eggs on a candida cleanse and diet unless you have serious cholesterol issues. You can always use egg whites if you need to without negatively impacting your cleanse. Eggs will keep you going all morning and are a quick way to get a hot, satisfying meal.

- 2 tablespoons olive oil
- ½ small onion, chopped
- ½ red pepper, chopped
- Any other veggies you like that are on your list
- 2 to 3 eggs, beaten
- Sea salt, black pepper, and paprika to taste
- Handful of fresh spinach

1. Heat a skillet and add the olive oil. Cook the onions until translucent.

2. Add the pepper and cook about 1 to 2 minutes more; you want the pepper tender but not mushy.

3. Add seasonings to beaten eggs and stir in. Set aside.

4. Add the spinach to the other veggies when they are done and cook only until wilted.

5. Pour the beaten eggs over the veggies and cook until done. Turn omelet over and serve immediately.

Buckwheat Hot Cereal

Makes 1 Serving

Toasted buckwheat groats are also known as kasha and may be sold that way, but make sure there is nothing else in them if you purchase them that way. To toast buckwheat groats, place them in a dry pan over medium heat, stirring, for 5 minutes, until browned. Toasting gives them a nice, nutty flavor.

- ½ cup buckwheat groats, toasted
- 1 cup water for cooking
- 2 tablespoons coconut oil
- Coconut milk for serving
- Ground cinnamon
- Stevia

---

1. Put groats and cooking water into a pot and bring to a boil. Reduce heat to low and simmer for 15 to 20 minutes. Drain the water; then stir in the coconut milk and oil.

2. Mix in cinnamon and stevia to taste. Garnish if you like with nuts, coconut, or other extras that are on your list.

Coconut Granola Parfait

Makes 1 Serving

In the mood for something cool and creamy? A yogurt-based breakfast is packed with protein and probiotics. You're doing yourself a favor with this kind of start to the day.

- 1 cup plain yogurt
- Stevia to taste
- 1 cup (or more if you're really hungry) coconut
- Granola (recipe on page 69)
- Nuts, seeds, coconut, and any other safe garnish you like

Sweeten the yogurt if you like. In a large glass, layer the granola with the yogurt. Garnish as you see fit.

Avocado Omelet

Makes 1 Serving

Avocado is a one of the major power foods on the candida cleanse, and teamed up with eggs it's unbeatable. You get a lot of energy from this omelet, so don't be afraid to plan a lot of activities on a day you start this way.

- 3 eggs
- Sea salt, black pepper, and paprika to taste
- 2 tablespoons chopped fresh parsley, divided
- 1 tablespoon butter
- 2 shallots, chopped
- 2 cloves garlic, chopped
- 1 avocado, halved and sliced
- 6 to 7 black olives (not the ones in vinegar)

1. Beat the eggs in a bowl with salt, pepper, paprika, and ¾ of the parsley. Set aside.

2. Melt the butter in a nonstick skillet over medium heat. Sauté the shallots and garlic until slightly browned. Remove the shallots and garlic from the pan and set them aside, but do not clean the pan.

3. Add the egg mixture to the pan and let it cook for 3 to 4 minutes, or until omelet is solid. Turn over once, and remove omelet from pan.

4. Spread the shallots and garlic evenly over the omelet. Add the avocado slices, olives, and the remaining parsley, fold over, and serve.

Eggs and Turkey Not-Sausage

Makes 1 Serving

While processed meats are off the candida-safe list, you can make your own substitutes that taste better and make you feel great. Spices and excellent quality meats are the key.

- Roasted turkey slices, about 1 pound
- Sea salt, ground sage, fennel seed (optional) to taste
- 1 egg, beaten
- Olive oil for oiling skillet
- 3 eggs, cooked to order

1. Using a food processor or blender, grind up all ingredients except the eggs. Process to a coarse grind. Transfer to a bowl and mix in the 1 beaten egg.

2. Shape into patties and chill for a minimum of 1 hour.

3. Cook in oiled skillet until crispy on each side and serve hot. (You don't need to worry about how long you cook these, as the meat was precooked.) Serve with the eggs cooked to order.

Breakfast Sandwich

Makes 1 Serving

Busy? Take your breakfast with you.

- 2 slices Spinach Bread (recipe on page 138)
- 1 egg, fried or scrambled
- 1 tomato slice
- 2 avocado slices
- 2 to 3 leaves baby spinach
- 1 piece Turkey Not-Sausage (recipe on page 56), or you may use any meat you like
- Any sauce or dressing from this book
- Breakfast seasoning from this book or other seasoning to taste

---

Layer ingredients to make a sandwich and enjoy.

Rhubarb Yogurt Parfait

Makes 1 Serving

Breakfast doesn't always have to be the same old thing. Create a beautiful, colorful parfait for yourself and get fired up for the day. Or eat a food you haven't tried for years and wake up your taste buds along with the rest of you.

- 1 rhubarb stalk, peeled and chopped into small pieces
- ½ tablespoon butter
- Stevia to taste
- Dash arrowroot powder
- 1 cup Greek yogurt
- Shredded, unsweetened coconut

---

1. In a small saucepan cook rhubarb, butter, stevia, and arrowroot until rhubarb mixture is slightly thickened and sweet enough for you. Cool.

2. Layer with yogurt and coconut, and serve.

6

SNACKS (CLEANSE)

Whenever you're trying something new, especially a cleanse and diet as challenging as this one, you're going to need some snacks to get you through the day. This program definitely has you covered. The candida-free lifestyle truly does offer you a wide variety of exciting options.

In this chapter:

Grilled Fennel Dippers

Coconut Bread

Guacamole

Macadamia Nut "Hummus"

Tzatziki

Sardine Pâté

Onion Herb Crackers

Lemony Kale Chips

Coconut Granola

Grilled Fennel Dippers

Makes 2 Servings

This is one of the most innovative and delicious snacks in the book, and it's simple as can be. Even if you've never had it, try it—it will quickly be high on your list. Fennel goes with just about any of the dips, sauces, and dressings offered in this diet.

- 1 fennel bulb, sliced into triangles
- Seasonings to taste

- 1 batch Macadamia Nut Hummus (recipe on page 63), Guacamole (recipe on page 62), or other dip in this book

---

1. Preheat your indoor or outdoor grill.

2. In order to slice your fennel bulb to make the perfect dipper, cut it in half vertically and then remove the core by cutting a triangle into the base of each half bulb. Then peel off layers as if the fennel were an onion, and slice these layers into triangles (or at least shapes you can handle).

3. Place fennel slices on the grill and sprinkle with whatever safe seasonings you like. Close the top and allow to cook for 2 to 3 minutes. The fennel should still be crisp.

4. Serve with dip of your choice.

Coconut Bread

Makes 1 Loaf

And you thought bread was off the menu. It's true that most commercial breads are off your list. But when you give these breads a try, you are going to be pleasantly surprised, not only with the way they taste, but also with how easy they are to make.

- 5 eggs
- 2 tablespoons coconut oil, and for greasing pan
- Stevia to taste
- ½ teaspoon sea salt
- ½ cup coconut flour
- ½ cup buckwheat flour
- ½ cup coconut milk (use only the creamy part on the top)
- 1 teaspoon baking powder

1. Preheat oven to 350°F. Blend the eggs, coconut oil, stevia, and salt in a large bowl.

2. Add the coconut flour, buckwheat flour, coconut milk, and baking powder, and whisk until you don't see any lumps.

3. Pour into a loaf pan greased with coconut oil and bake for 30 minutes. The top of the loaf should be firm and a light golden color. Remove from the oven and allow to cool.

Guacamole

Makes About 2 Cups

Another delicious way to take advantage of the healthful fats in avocado is also a universal party favorite. This is easy as can be and will fill you up—not to mention keep your friends happy.

- 2 avocados, chopped
- ½ onion, grated
  (it becomes a pulp)
- 1 clove garlic, grated
- Fresh lemon juice to taste
- Minced cilantro to taste, plus extra sprigs for garnish
- Sea salt and white pepper to taste

Put all the ingredients in a bowl and mash them up thoroughly. Serve with a garnish of cilantro on top.

Macadamia Nut "Hummus"

Makes About 2 Cups

Feeling that afternoon drag? You need a quick fix with protein and a great energy source, just like this.

- 1 cup macadamia nuts
- 1 large tomato
- 1/3 cup fresh basil leaves
- 1 clove garlic, peeled
- 1/2 teaspoon cayenne pepper
- Juice of 1/2 lemon
- Sea salt to taste

1. Soak the macadamia nuts in water for about 2 hours. Drain.

2. Steam or roast the tomato until slightly soft.

3. In a food processor or blender, combine all ingredients and blend until smooth. Chill.

Tzatziki

Makes About 2 Cups

This traditional Greek dip can feel like a mini meal in itself when you serve it with cucumbers or candida-safe breads or crackers for dipping. This satisfying snack option is packed with protein and flavor.

- 1 cup plain yogurt
- ½ cucumber, peeled and diced
- 1 clove garlic, minced
- 1 teaspoon apple cider vinegar
- 1 teaspoon chopped fresh dill
- 1 tablespoon olive oil
- Sea salt and white pepper to taste

Mix all ingredients in a bowl and refrigerate for at least 1 hour for the best flavor.

Sardine Pâté

Makes About 1½ Cups

Sardines may sound like a punch line instead of something delicious that can make a wonderful appetizer, but give this a try. You are going to be impressed.

- 12 ounces boneless sardines in oil, drained
- 1 clove garlic
- 2 shallots, peeled
- 1 tablespoon butter
- 2 tablespoons chopped fresh parsley
- ½ bunch fresh chives
- Juice of ½ lemon
- Dash of black pepper

Blend all ingredients in a food processor or blender until smooth. Serve with candida-safe crackers like Onion Herb Crackers (recipe on page 66), vegetable crudités, or other treats.

Onion Herb Crackers

Makes 2 Large Sheets of Crackers

Once you give these crispy treats a try, you'll want to keep them on hand all the time. A perfect fallback option for candida sufferers, they go great with just about everything.

- 1 cup coarsely chopped sweet onion, such as Vidalia
- 1 large clove garlic, minced
- ¼ cup grape-seed oil
- 2 teaspoons fresh thyme leaves
- ¼ teaspoon Himalayan rock salt or sea salt
- Coarsely ground black pepper to taste
- 1½ cups roughly ground flaxseeds or milled flaxseeds
- ¼ cup finely ground sunflower seeds

1. Preheat oven to 225°F. Set out two large baking sheets.

2. Pulse onion, garlic, oil, thyme, salt, and pepper in a food processor until onion is completely puréed.

3. Add flaxseeds and sunflower seeds, and pulse just until combined. Transfer to a large bowl.

4. Roll about ½ cup of the cracker dough into a ball and place it in the middle of a piece of parchment paper about 12 inches wide. Fold the paper like a book with the ball between the "covers," and then roll the dough between them until it's about ¼ inch thick.

5. Unfold or tear away the top half of the paper. Score the crackers into 1-inch squares. Keeping the crackers on their current sheet of parchment, transfer the sheet to a baking sheet. Repeat with remaining dough.

6. Bake for 2 hours, flipping halfway through and removing the top layer of parchment paper after you've flipped the dough over. The baking time will vary greatly on how thin you make the crackers. The end result should be crisp and crunchy with no moisture left.

7. Remove from the oven and allow to cool on the baking sheet for 15 minutes before storing in an airtight container.

Lemony Kale Chips

Makes 2–3 Servings

Crispy, crunchy, and full of vitamins, kale chips are a wonderful snack for anyone, but they are irreplaceable for this candida regimen.

- 1 bunch kale, larger stem pieces removed
- 2 tablespoons olive oil
- 2 tablespoons fresh lemon juice
- ¼ teaspoon sea salt

---

1. Preheat oven to 350°F. Chop kale into ½-inch pieces. Place kale in a large bowl and work all other ingredients into the kale with your fingers.

2. Place chips on a parchment-lined baking sheet and bake at 350°F for 10 to 15 minutes. The kale should be dark green and crispy, but be very careful to avoid burning.

3. Cool and serve. Store in an airtight container.

Coconut Granola

Makes 3 Cups

Perfect for snack time or breakfast, this granola is sweet and delicious. In case you have a sweet-tooth emergency, reach for something that won't throw your system out of whack.

- 1 cup oat bran
- 1 cup buckwheat groats, toasted
- ½ cup chia seeds
- ¼ cup coconut oil
- 2 teaspoons stevia
- 2 tablespoons ground cinnamon
- Sea salt to taste
- ½ cup unsweetened, shredded coconut

---

1. Preheat the oven to 300°F. In a large bowl mix all the ingredients except the shredded coconut. Make certain that everything is well coated with coconut oil.

2. Spread the mixture evenly on a baking sheet lined with parchment paper and bake for 12 minutes.

3. Add the coconut and stir, turning the granola so it browns evenly. Bake for another 12 minutes.

4. Store in an airtight container.

7

SOUPS, SALADS, SANDWICHES, AND SIDES (CLEANSE)

S pice up your menu with these diverse side dishes. Whether you're in the mood for something light like a salad or it's a chilly day and nothing will do but soup, the recipes in this chapter have you covered. Try fun treats like Jicama Fries.

In this chapter:

Beef Stock

Even if you've never done it, you absolutely need to start to make your own stock. It's the key to making candida-safe recipes, because almost any soup, dressing, or sauce you buy commercially has additives that can contribute to the overgrowth problem.

- Olive oil
- 1 pound stew meat (chuck or flank steak) and/or beef scraps, cut into 2-inch chunks
- 1 to 2 medium onions, peeled and quartered
- 4 to 5 pounds meaty beef stock bones (with lots of marrow), including some knuckle bones, cut to expose the center marrow
- 2 or 3 veal bones if available
- Handful of celery tops or 1 large celery rib cut into 1-inch segments
- 2 to 3 cloves garlic, unpeeled
- Handful of fresh parsley stems and leaves
- 1 to 2 bay leaves
- 10 peppercorns

1. Preheat oven to 400°F. Rub a little olive oil over the stew meat pieces and onions.

2. Place stock bones, stew meat or beef scraps, and onions in a large, shallow roasting pan. Roast in the oven for about 45 minutes, turning the bones and meat pieces halfway through the cooking, until nicely browned. If bones begin to char during this cooking process, lower the heat. They should brown, not burn.

3. When the bones and meat are nicely browned, remove them and the onions and place them in a large (12–16 quart) stock pot.

4. Place the roasting pan on the stove top on low heat. It will cover two burners. Pour ½ to 1 cup hot water over the pan and use a metal spatula

to scrape up all the browned bits stuck to the bottom of the pan. Pour the browned bits and water into the stock pot.

5. Add celery tops, garlic, parsley, bay leaves, and peppercorns to the stock pot. Fill the stock pot with cold water to 1 to 2 inches over the top of the bones.

6. Put the heat on high and bring the pot to a low simmer; then reduce the heat to low. If you have a candy or meat thermometer, the temperature of the water should be between 180°F and 200°F (boiling is 212°F). The stock should be at a bare simmer, just a bubble or two coming up here and there. (You may need to put the pot on your smallest burner on the lowest temp, or if you are using an oven-safe pot, place it in the oven at 190°F.)

7. Cover the pot loosely and let simmer low and slow for 3 to 6 hours. Do not stir the stock while cooking. Stirring will mix the fats in with the stock, clouding up the stock.

8. As the stock cooks, fat will be released from the bone marrow and stew meat and rise to the top. From time to time check in on the stock and use a large metal spoon to scoop away the fat and any scum that rises to the surface. (Do not put this fat down your kitchen drain. It will solidify and block your pipes. Put it in a bowl or jar to save for cooking or to discard.)

9. At the end of cooking time, use tongs or a slotted spoon to gently remove the bones and vegetables from the pot. Discard them; though if you see a chunk of marrow, taste it—it's delicious.

10. Pour the stock through a fine-mesh sieve lined with two layers of cheesecloth, into a large clean pot (about 8 quarts). Let cool to room temperature; then chill in the refrigerator.

11. Once the stock has chilled, any fat remaining will rise to the top and solidify. The fat forms a protective layer against bacteria while the stock is in the refrigerator. If you plan to freeze the stock, however, remove and discard the fat and pour the stock into a jar or plastic container. (You can also remove the fat and boil the stock down, concentrating it so that it doesn't take as much storage space.) Leave 1 inch of head room from the top of the stock to the top of the jar so that as the stock freezes and expands, it will not break the container.

Chicken Stock

Once you start making and using your own stock, you'll see how easy it is, and you can readily keep it on hand. Give it a try, perhaps with this chicken stock, which is simple to make. The first method uses leftover bones and the second uses fresh chicken pieces.

Method 1: Leftover chicken bones

- Leftover bones and skin from a cooked or raw chicken carcass
- Celery (at least one stalk)
- Onions (at least one), cut in quarters
- ½ cup fresh parsley
- Sea salt and black pepper to taste

---

1. Put everything into a large stock pot and cover with cold water. Bring to a boil and immediately reduce heat to bring the stock to a bare simmer. Simmer uncovered for at least 4 hours (longer is better), occasionally skimming off the foam that comes to the surface.

2. Remove the bones and strain the stock.

Method 2: Chicken backs, wings, and legs

- 1 large yellow onion, chopped
- 1 tablespoon olive oil
- 4 pounds chicken backs, wings, and legs, cut into 2-inch pieces (ask your butcher or meat counter to do this)
- 2 quarts boiling water
- 2 teaspoons sea salt
- 2 bay leaves

1. Heat 1 tablespoon olive oil in a large stock pot. Add onion. Sauté until softened and slightly colored, about 2 to 3 minutes.

2. Add the chicken parts, bay leaves, and salt to the stock pot and pour in boiling water. Proceed as described in Method 1.

Vegetable Stock

You don't need to be a vegetarian to enjoy vegetable stock. You can make this in minutes and use it in place of any kind of stock.

- 2 medium onions, chopped
- 1 large handful of kale or chard, chopped
- 4 stalks celery, chopped
- 3 cloves garlic
- Sea salt and cayenne pepper to taste
- Fresh dill to taste

Place ingredients in 2 quarts water. Bring to boil and simmer for 20 minutes; then strain the liquid and discard the veggies. If you'd like to spice it up a little, throw in some cayenne pepper. This is the minimum simmer time; longer is better, and you can simmer for several hours if you like—up to 6 or 7, though this isn't necessary.

Gazpacho

Makes 3–4 Servings

Think cold soup sounds just wrong? Did you think of iced coffee that way the first time you heard of it, or iced tea? Try these cold soup recipes for a refreshing treat.

- 3–4 tomatoes
- ½ cucumber
- 1 bell pepper (any color)
- 1 shallot
- 1 clove garlic
- ½ cup cilantro
- Juice of 2 limes
- 1 tablespoon apple cider vinegar
- 2 tablespoons olive oil
- 1 cup water
- ½ tablespoon red chili flakes
- Sea salt and black pepper to taste

1. Core the tomatoes. Blanch and peel the tomatoes. Next dice the tomatoes and put them in a food processor or blender.

2. Set aside about one-third each of the cucumber and bell pepper.

3. Add the remaining ingredients to the food processor and blend with the tomatoes until smooth.

4. Chop the reserved bell pepper and cucumber and stir them in the soup. Sprinkle with extra chili flakes and serve.

Broccoli Soup

Makes About 2 Quarts

This is comfort food at its finest, and healthful to boot. Don't wait for winter.

- 2 tablespoons olive oil
- 1 medium onion, chopped
- 1 bunch broccoli, coarsely chopped
- 2 quarts stock or water
- ½ teaspoon sea salt

In a large pot over medium-low heat, sauté the onion in the oil until soft. Add broccoli and sauté for 5 to 10 minutes. Add water and cook until broccoli is soft, about 15 minutes. Purée hot soup in small batches using a food processor or blender on high until smooth and creamy.

Avocado Cucumber Gazpacho

Makes About 3 Cups

This soup is wonderfully creamy and flavorful, but still light. You will love this riff on the traditional Spanish version.

- 2 large avocados
- ½ cucumber
- ¼ onion
- ½ cup plain yogurt
- 2 cloves garlic
- 1½ cups cold stock or water
- Sea salt and black pepper to taste

1. Scoop out the avocado flesh. Chop up the cucumber and onion into large pieces.

2. Purée avocado, cucumber, onion, yogurt, garlic, water, and seasonings in a food processor or blender. Chill and serve.

Soba Seaweed Salad

Makes 2 Servings

You'll love the way soba noodles fill you up but don't weigh you down, and you'll be amazed at the many health benefits you glean from seaweed. This is one for almost any diet.

- ¼ cup shredded dry seaweed (make sure it passes the label test)
- 2 tomatoes
- 1 avocado

- 2 ounces soba noodles, cooked according to directions on package
- 2 tablespoons sesame oil
- Sprinkle of sesame seeds
- Sea salt to taste

1. Soak the seaweed in a bowl of warm water for about 10 minutes. Drain.

2. Chop the tomatoes and avocado; then put seaweed, tomatoes, avocado, and soba noodles into a large bowl and mix. Drizzle with sesame oil and sprinkle with the sesame seeds. Serve cold.

Quinoa Tabbouleh

Makes 4 Servings

Quinoa is loaded with protein, and this cold dish is something you can keep in the fridge and eat whenever you like. You'll love how versatile this dish is, as a side, snack, or small meal.

- ½ cup uncooked quinoa, rinsed
- 3 cups finely minced fresh parsley
- ½ cup finely minced fresh mint leaves
- 10 cherry tomatoes, chopped
- ½ cucumber, chopped
- 1 red onion, chopped
- ½ cup fresh lemon juice
- 3 tablespoons olive oil
- Sea salt and black pepper to taste

1. Cook quinoa as directed in stock or water. Cool.

2. Mix all the ingredients well and chill. Flavor is best if it can chill for at least 1 hour after mixing.

Spicy Slaw

Makes 2 Servings

Put a little kick into your afternoon with some spice. Herbs and spices will save you from monotony on the candida cleanse, and they will also help your digestive system back to a state of good health.

- ½ head purple cabbage, shredded
- 1 bunch cilantro, finely chopped
- 1 jalapeño pepper, seeded and minced
- 1 teaspoon minced fresh ginger
- Juice of 2 limes
- 2 tablespoons olive oil
- 7 drops stevia
- ½ teaspoon sea salt

1. Place the cabbage, cilantro, jalapeño, and ginger in a large bowl.

2. Toss with lime juice, olive oil, and stevia; then sprinkle with salt. Serve.

Sautéed Wilted Kale Salad

Makes 2 Servings

Yet another amazing use for kale, this recipe proves that simpler is often better. Caramelized onions give it tremendous flavor.

- 2 tablespoons olive oil
- 1 medium onion, chopped
- 1 bunch kale, trimmed and chopped into 1-inch strips, thick center stems discarded
- ¼ teaspoon sea salt

---

1. In a large pan, heat oil over medium heat. Reduce heat to medium-low and add onion. Sauté onion for 15 minutes, or until caramelized.

2. Add kale and sauté for 5 minutes. Cover pot with a lid and cook for 1 to 2 minutes, or until kale is wilted. Add sea salt and serve.

Grilled Lime Chicken Sandwich

Makes 1 Sandwich

Sometimes there's no substitute for a sandwich, and even though commercial breads are off the menu, sandwiches definitely aren't. The marinated chicken in this sandwich is packed with protein and taste.

- Juice of 2 limes
- 3 cloves garlic
- 2 mild chiles of your choice
- 1 tablespoon olive oil
- Sea salt and black pepper to taste

- 1 chicken breast
- Your choice of Coconut Bread (recipe on page 61), Spinach Bread (recipe on page 138), or Basic Candida-Safe Bread (recipe on page 222)

1. In a food processor or blender, purée the lime juice, garlic, chiles, olive oil, salt, and pepper. Pour into a resealable plastic bag with the chicken breast. Seal the bag and let it marinate in the refrigerator for 30–60 minutes.

2. Grill the chicken until it's cooked thoroughly, or if you don't have access to a grill, cook it in a hot, lightly oiled skillet.

3. Serve on Coconut Bread, Spinach Bread, or Basic Candida-Safe Bread.

Turkey Zucchini Burger

Makes 5–6 Burgers

If you're missing things like burgers and fries, stop missing them. Make them the right way for yourself.

- 1 pound turkey breast fillets
- 1 cup chopped zucchini
- 1-inch piece fresh ginger, peeled and chopped
- 2 spring onions, chopped
- ¼ cup chopped fresh cilantro
- 1 tablespoon coconut aminos
- 1 egg
- 3 tablespoons ground flaxseeds
- Coconut oil
- Your choice of Coconut Bread (recipe on page 61), Spinach Bread (recipe on page 138), or Basic Candida-Safe Bread (recipe on page 222)

1. Using a food processor or blender, process everything except the coconut oil until it reaches a good patty consistency.

2. Heat the oil in a large frying pan over medium-high heat. Form five or six patties and cook them for 3 to 4 minutes on each side, or until browned and cooked thoroughly.

3. Serve on Coconut Bread, Spinach Bread, or Basic Candida-Safe Bread.

No-Potato Salad

Makes 4 Servings

The picnic classic can be revamped for candida sufferers, and this recipe does it. Take care to stay close to the stove while you cook the cauliflower so you don't overcook it.

- 1 head cauliflower, broken into small florets
- 2 stalks celery, diced
- 1 small onion, finely chopped
- 1 tablespoon finely chopped fresh parsley
- 2 eggs, hard boiled and diced

- 2 tablespoons homemade Mayonnaise (recipe on page 211)
- 1 teaspoon dry mustard
- 1 teaspoon apple cider vinegar
- ½ teaspoon sea salt

1. Steam cauliflower on the stove until just fork-tender. If overcooked, a strong "cauliflower" smell develops. Allow cauliflower to cool, then place in a large bowl.

2. Add celery, onion, parsley, and egg. Stir in mayonnaise, mustard, apple cider vinegar, and salt. Chill and serve.

Jicama Fries

Makes 6 Servings

Get ready to start loving jicama. Jicama is one of the lowest-calorie root vegetables, at only 250 calories per medium jicama—usually almost 3 cups. One of the finest sources of dietary fiber and high in antioxidants, jicama also contains respectable proportions of minerals and vitamins. It is an excellent source of oligofructose inulin, which is a zero-calorie, sweet-inert carbohydrate, and soluble dietary fiber, which does not metabolize in the human body. This makes jicama an ideal sweet snack for people with diabetes and candida sufferers.

- 1 jicama, skin removed and sliced into thin strips
- ½ teaspoon olive oil
- 1 teaspoon paprika
- ½ teaspoon onion powder
- Pinch of salt
- Pinch of cayenne (optional)

1. Toss all ingredients together in a large bowl until fries are well coated.

2. Fry in your choice of oil or bake at 400°F for 25 minutes, turning fries and pan halfway through baking time.

Oven-Roasted Asparagus

Makes 2 Servings

This one is so simple, it's practically not a recipe—but the results say otherwise. This goes wonderfully with just about everything.

- 1 bunch asparagus, tough ends trimmed and discarded

- 2 tablespoons olive oil
- ¼ to ½ teaspoon sea salt

---

1. Preheat oven to 350°F. Lay asparagus spears side by side in a single layer in a 9-by-13-inch baking dish lined with parchment paper. Drizzle with olive oil and sprinkle with sea salt.

2. Give the pan a few shakes to roll the asparagus a half-turn. Roast in the oven for 10 to 12 minutes; remove from oven when tips start to brown. Cool a few minutes, and then serve.

8

MAIN DISHES (CLEANSE)

If you were ever worried about your new anti-candida regimen resulting in your table being bare, hopefully this chapter will put those worries to rest forever.

In this chapter:

Steak with Ginger Sauce

Makes 1 Serving

This dish tastes so wonderful you won't even remember it's on your cleanse diet. Adjust the level of ginger for your own personal taste.

- 1 steak of your choice
- Seasonings of your choice
- ¼ cup grated fresh ginger
- 4 cloves garlic, chopped
- Coconut aminos (as a substitute for soy sauce)
- Chili powder to taste
- Juice of 1 lemon
- Olive oil as needed for dressing

---

1. Season and cook the steak to your liking.

2. While the steak is cooking, make the sauce: Mix together the grated ginger, garlic, coconut aminos, chili powder, lemon juice, and enough olive oil to make a dressing. Adjust seasonings and serve the steak sliced, drizzled with the sauce.

Tandoori Chicken or Lamb

Makes 4 Servings

One of the best ways to succeed with the candida cleanse and diet is by making the most of herbs and spices. You can do so much with them to keep your food interesting. The curries and sauces presented in this book give you some great places to start.

- Cubed uncooked chicken or lamb to serve 4
- ¼ cup coconut milk
- Juice of ½ lemon
- 2 teaspoons minced garlic
- 2 teaspoons grated fresh ginger
- 2 teaspoons ground cumin
- ½ teaspoon ground coriander
- ¼ teaspoon cayenne pepper
- ⅛ teaspoon ground cloves
- ⅛ teaspoon black pepper
- Pinch of sea salt
- Pinch of ground cardamom
- 2 sliced onions and other vegetables of your choice for roasting and serving

---

1. Place cubed chicken or lamb in a glass container. Set aside.

2. Combine the rest of the ingredients except the onions and vegetables, and stir thoroughly. Pour over the meat. Mix with a spoon, seal with a lid, and marinate in the fridge for 8 to 48 hours. More time adds more flavor.

3. When you are ready to cook, preheat oven to 375°F and line two baking sheets with parchment paper. Place marinated meat cubes on one of the sheets, spacing them to allow them to cook evenly.

4. Toss vegetables with olive oil, salt, and pepper, and place on the other baking sheet.

5. Put both pans into oven to roast. If the vegetables are done first, remove them and pop them back in the oven at the end for a few minutes to warm them.

6. Turn the pieces at least once during the cooking time. Bake until the meat is cooked through; split a larger piece to check. Remove from the oven when done and allow to sit.

7. Serve the meat over the vegetables.

Cabbage Masala

Makes 3–4 Servings

Don't back away from cabbage, and the same goes for Indian spices. Once you give recipes like this a try, you'll love the variety they provide in your routine. Garam masala is a traditional Indian spice mixture that generally contains only spices allowable on the candida cleanse and diet—read the label to make sure.

- 3 tablespoons coconut oil
- 1 teaspoon yellow mustard seeds , or 1/2 teaspoon mustard powder
- 5 cloves garlic, minced
- 1 large onion, yellow or white, sliced very thin
- ¼ teaspoon ground turmeric
- 1 teaspoon garam masala
- 1 teaspoon ground cumin
- 2 large tomatoes, finely sliced
- ¾ cup sliced okra
- ½ head green cabbage, sliced
- 1 teaspoon sea salt

1. Heat oil in a large skillet and add the mustard seeds. (If you use mustard powder, add it with the spices in Step 3.) Once they pop, add the garlic and cook until slightly soft.

2. Add the onion and cook until soft.

3. Add the turmeric, garam masala, and cumin, and cook for another 2 to 3 minutes.

4. Add the tomatoes and okra, cover, and cook for 5 minutes.

5. Add the cabbage and salt. Cook for a further 15 minutes. Serve hot.

Coconut Chicken with Spinach

Makes 2 Servings

This hearty dish is packed with nutty flavor and protein. The spinach and coconut work especially well together.

- ½ cup almonds
- 3 tablespoons coconut oil
- ½ cup coconut milk
- 3 cups baby spinach
- 1 large onion, chopped
- 1 large chicken breast, cubed
- Sea salt and black pepper to taste

1. Pulse the almonds in a food processor until they are coarsely chopped; then lightly brown them in a pan with coconut oil. Set aside.

2. Place coconut milk and spinach into a small saucepan on low heat. Cover and simmer for about 3 minutes.

3. In a large skillet sauté the onions until translucent. Add chicken to the onions and cook thoroughly.

4. Add coconut milk and spinach to the chicken and onions. Stir and cover. Let simmer about 2 to 3 minutes so flavors mingle.

5. Serve topped with toasted almonds, salt, and pepper.

Asparagus with Anchovies and Soba Noodles

Makes 1–2 Servings

There is almost no food more unfairly maligned than the lowly anchovy. Chances are excellent that you've had them before and didn't know it. They are a common ingredient in Worcestershire sauce, other prepared fish sauces, many Caesar salad dressings, tapenades, and green goddess dressings. Anchovies provide a salty, nutty quality, and when they are cooked down into a sauce or dish they are flavorful and rich, but mild. Anchovies are also full of fatty acids that can help lower cholesterol and reduce heart disease. And anchovies are a great (and sustainable) source of protein, calcium, and vitamins E and D.

- 5 ounces soba noodles
- 2 tablespoons butter
- 10 asparagus spears, tough ends removed
- 20–30 flat anchovy fillets in olive oil
- 3 cloves garlic, chopped
- 1 mild chile (Anaheim works well), seeded and chopped

1. Cook soba noodles in water as directed on the package. Drain and set aside.

2. Heat butter in a shallow, wide skillet and add the garlic, chile, anchovies, and asparagus. Cover with a lid and let cook for 8 to 10 minutes. Add the soba noodles, toss, and season to taste.

Quinoa Meatloaf

Makes 4 Servings

This is a great one to make in a hurry by using whatever leftover meat you have out of the fridge and coupling it with quinoa. And who says a nice slice of leftover meatloaf can't be breakfast or a snack?

- ¼ cup uncooked quinoa, rinsed
- 1 pound cooked turkey, chicken, lamb, or beef, minced
- 2 eggs, beaten
- 1 medium onion, finely chopped
- 3 cloves garlic, minced
- 1 teaspoon coconut oil or olive oil, and for oiling pan
- 1 teaspoon dried thyme
- 1 teaspoon dried rosemary
- ¼ teaspoon black pepper
- 1 teaspoon sea salt
- Chili powder to taste
- Paprika to taste

1. Preheat oven to 350°F. Cook quinoa as directed (with homemade stock if you can).

2. Mix the cooked quinoa and all other ingredients in a large bowl.

3. Oil a loaf pan, add the mixture, and bake for 1 hour.

Cabbage Rolls

Makes 2–3 Servings

This traditional dish might not be the way Grandma made it, but it's even better. No offense to Grandma, but when you use organic meat and mince it yourself, you're going to love it even more.

- 1 head green cabbage
- 1 pound organic boneless beef or lamb, minced (mince it yourself—no ground meats)
- ½ cup buckwheat groats, toasted
- 1 egg, beaten
- 2 medium onions, chopped
- 4 cloves garlic, minced
- 4 tomatoes, chopped
- 2 tablespoons olive oil
- Sea salt to taste

---

1. Preheat the oven to 350°F. Tear 6 to 8 leaves off the cabbage and steam until wilted enough to be flexible. Set aside to cool.

2. Put the meat, uncooked buckwheat groats, 1 of the chopped onions, egg, salt, and 2 of the minced garlic cloves into a large bowl. Mix thoroughly.

3. Roll the meat and buckwheat mixture up into the cabbage leaves.

4. For the tomato sauce, sauté the other onion and the remaining garlic in a wide, deep saucepan until onion is soft, about 10 minutes. Add chopped tomatoes and simmer for 5 to 10 minutes more.

5. Place the stuffed cabbage leaves in a 9-by-9-inch baking dish, either lined with parchment paper or oiled, and drizzle the rolls with the tomato sauce. Add ½ cup water and cover with foil.

6. Bake in the oven for 1 hour. Check under foil several times; add more water as needed.

7. Remove from oven and cool slightly. Serve with a dollop of plain yogurt.

Chicken Quinoa Chopped Dinner Salad

Makes 2 Servings

Quinoa is your friend when candida is your enemy. Quinoa is a pseudocereal, not a real grain, and it is also a complete source of protein. It's also a fantastic side dish and can stand in handsomely for rice, potatoes, and other starchy foes.

- 1 chicken breast, sliced or cubed
- 1 clove garlic, minced
- 2 tablespoons olive oil
- ⅔ cup cooked quinoa
- 2 cups coarsely chopped spinach
- 1 hard-boiled egg, sliced

- 2 medium tomatoes, coarsely chopped
- ½ cucumber, chopped
- 1 avocado, chopped
- 2 shallots, sliced
- Juice of ½ lemon
- Sea salt to taste

---

1. Heat oil in a broad, shallow skillet. Add garlic and chicken and cook until chicken is completely done. Cool chicken.

2. Put the chicken and remaining ingredients into a large bowl, toss to dress, and serve.

Beef and Okra Stew

Makes 2 Servings

You don't have to be in the Deep South to enjoy okra. This stew is more than a satisfying meal—it's a boost to your immune system, too.

- 1 large onion, in about four pieces
- 4–6 cloves garlic, peeled
- 2 chiles, seeded
- ½ pound cubed stew beef
- 3 tablespoons cooking oil of your choice
- 3 tomatoes, chopped
- 1 cup water
- ½ teaspoon cayenne pepper
- ¼ teaspoon cumin
- ¼ teaspoon black pepper
- 1 teaspoon sea salt
- ½ pound okra (cut crosswise with stems removed)

1. Process onion, garlic, and chiles in food processor until they form a paste.

2. Cook the meat in cooking oil in a large, deep saucepan for 2 to 3 minutes until lightly browned.

3. Add the paste and cook for another 2–3 minutes.

4. Add the tomatoes, water, spices, and seasoning and bring to a boil. Reduce the heat, add the okra, and simmer for 10 minutes.

Chipotle Lime Salmon

Makes 4 Servings

This dish is easy to prepare, and you can spice it up as much as you like. Add some omega fish oils to your life.

- 1 pound salmon, cut into 4 fillets
- 1 to 2 tablespoons olive oil
- 2 limes, sliced in half
- 1 teaspoon sea salt
- 1 teaspoon chipotle powder

1. Preheat oven to 450°F. Cover baking sheet with parchment paper.

2. Rub each fillet with olive oil.

3. Sprinkle fillets with salt and chipotle, then place a squeezed lime half on top of each fillet.

4. Bake the salmon in the oven for 10 to 18 minutes, depending on how well done you like your fish.

Roasted Chicken

Makes 4 Servings

This dish is perfect for serving guests even when you're in the middle of your candida cleanse. It's perfect for you and doesn't scrimp in any way for them.

- 1 whole chicken (2 to 3 pounds)
- Sea salt and black pepper to taste
- 1 bunch fresh thyme
- 1 lemon, halved
- 1 head garlic, cut in half crosswise
- 2 tablespoons olive oil
- 1 medium onion, quartered

---

1. Preheat oven to 425°F. Remove chicken giblets and rinse chicken inside and out. Pat chicken dry.

2. Place chicken in a 9-by-13-inch baking dish. Liberally salt and pepper inside of chicken.

3. Stuff cavity with the thyme, both halves of the lemon, and the garlic.

4. Brush the outside of the chicken with olive oil and sprinkle with salt and pepper.

5. Tie legs together with kitchen string and tuck wings under body of chicken. Place each onion quarter into a corner of dish.

6. Roast chicken for 1½ hours, or until its juices run clear. Allow to cool slightly and serve.

Herbed Salmon

Makes 4 Servings

Are you feeling like getting a little fancy? Why not sauce up some fresh, delicious salmon?

- 1 pound salmon
- 12 sprigs fresh thyme
- 12 sprigs fresh dill weed
- 1 tablespoon olive oil
- 1 teaspoon sea salt
- Black pepper to taste

1. Preheat oven to 450° F. Cover baking sheet with parchment paper.

2. Rub each fillet with olive oil. Place herbs underneath each fillet. Sprinkle fillets with salt and pepper.

3. Cook salmon in oven for 10 to 18 minutes, depending on how well done you like your fish. Serve with Leek Coulis or Herb Gravy (recipes on pages 218 and 109).

Veggies, Yogurt Cheese, and Quinoa

Makes 4 Servings

There are so many wonderful ways to use the homemade cheese you can make using the recipes in this book, and this way you avoid succumbing to your cravings. This dish is delicious and comforting.

- 3 bell peppers, chopped (different colors if possible)
- 6 to 10 shallots, peeled
- 6 to 10 cloves garlic, peeled
- 6 to 10 cherry tomatoes
- Olive oil
- Salt and black pepper to taste
- ½ cup uncooked quinoa, rinsed
- Handful of fresh basil leaves
- Juice of ½ lemon
- 1 tablespoon apple cider vinegar
- Homemade Yogurt Cheese (recipe on page 220)

1. Heat the oven to 450°F. Place peppers, shallots, garlic, and cherry tomatoes in an oiled roasting pan. Toss with the olive oil, salt, and pepper.

2. Spread in a single layer in the pan. Roast for 30 minutes, stirring occasionally, until the vegetables are lightly browned and tender.

3. Meanwhile, cook quinoa as directed, preferably with homemade stock.

4. Add the roasted vegetables and quinoa to a bowl. Toss with basil, lemon juice, and vinegar, and serve with crumbled yogurt cheese on top.

Grilled Asparagus Beef Rolls

Makes 4 Servings

This awesome meal can also stand in as a classy appetizer or dinner party offering. You'll love how quickly this comes together.

- 8–12 asparagus spears, with rough bottoms trimmed off
- ½ cup homemade Yogurt Cheese (recipe on page 220) or Almond Cheese (recipe on page 141)

- 4 pieces thinly sliced fresh beef
- 4 oil-packed sun-dried tomatoes
- 4 to 8 fresh basil leaves (depending on size)

1. Steam or boil the asparagus until just slightly tender and set aside.

2. Spread 2 tablespoons cheese on each slice of beef. Add a sun-dried tomato to each slice, plus 1 or 2 basil leaves.

3. Place 2 or 3 asparagus spears on top; then roll the beef around it. Stick a toothpick through each roll to hold it together.

4. Place on a preheated grill or in a frying pan for about 3 to 4 minutes on each side, or until beef is cooked.

Stuffed Peppers with Chicken and Quinoa

Makes 2 Servings

Beautiful, delicious, and safe for candida sufferers? Yes, please!

- ¼ cup uncooked quinoa, rinsed
- 3 tablespoons olive oil, divided
- 1 large onion, finely chopped
- 3 cloves garlic, minced
- 1 tomato, chopped
- ½ pound chicken breast meat, chopped
- 1 egg, lightly beaten
- 1 tablespoon dried basil
- 1 tablespoon dried parsley
- Sea salt, black pepper, and cayenne pepper to taste
- 2 red bell peppers, halved lengthwise

1. Preheat the oven to 350°F. Cook the quinoa as directed using homemade stock.

2. Heat 1 tablespoon olive oil in a large, deep skillet. Add onion and garlic to pan and sauté until translucent.

3. Add tomato and cook for 2 minutes more. Add the meat to the pan and cook until cooked through.

4. Combine all the ingredients except the red bell peppers and pack the mixture into the bell pepper halves. Bake for 30 minutes, or until peppers are tender.

Coconut Fried Chicken

Makes 24 Drumsticks

Coconut is amazing. It guards against heart disease, kills disease-causing bacteria and fungi including candida, slows the release of sugar into the bloodstream, helps prevent strokes and brain disorders such as Alzheimer's and Parkinson's, improves metabolism and boosts energy, and even prevents tooth decay. Plus, it's delicious with fried chicken.

- About 1 cup coconut oil, or enough for frying
- 1 cup coconut flour
- 1 teaspoon sea salt
- 1 teaspoon black pepper
- 1 cup coconut milk
- 1 egg, beaten
- 24 chicken drumsticks

---

1. Preheat oven to 300°F. Heat coconut oil in a large, deep frying pan until it starts to bubble and snaps if you sprinkle water on it.

2. Combine coconut flour, salt, and pepper in a dish. Beat coconut milk and egg together in another bowl.

3. One at a time, wet drumsticks with the coconut milk and egg mixture and shake off excess. Coat the drumsticks with the coconut flour mixture and put in the heated oil.

4. Repeat until pan is full. Let the drumsticks fry for about 5 to 8 minutes. Flip them over carefully with two forks and let them fry an additional 5–8 minutes. Repeat with remaining drumsticks.

5. Lay the fried drumsticks in a 9-by-13-inch baking pan (or two, if you need more space). Bake for about 1 to 1½ hours.

Pepper Steak with Herb Gravy

Makes 2 Servings

There are few things more satisfying than a nice hot meal with meat and gravy. Check out this revamp of an old classic.

- ½ cup coconut aminos, divided
- ½ teaspoon black pepper
- 2 steaks, any kind you like
- 1 cup beef stock (homemade only)
- ½ cup coconut aminos

- 2 tablespoons coconut oil
- 2 cloves garlic, minced
- 1 teaspoon minced fresh ginger
- 1 green bell pepper, julienned
- 1 medium onion, sliced

---

1. Combine coconut aminos and black pepper in a large resealable plastic bag. Place the steaks in the bag and seal. Turn the bag several times to coat the steaks and place bag in the refrigerator for 30 to 60 minutes.

2. In a medium-sized bowl combine beef stock and remaining ½ cup coconut aminos. Set aside.

3. Heat coconut oil in a deep skillet. Add garlic, ginger, green pepper, and onion, and sauté until the onion and bell pepper are crisp tender.

4. While you're sautéing, place the steaks under the broiler and cook on both sides until they are done to your liking.

5. For the gravy, add the stock-aminos mixture to the skillet with the vegetables and let it simmer over medium-low heat. Serve steaks topped with gravy and vegetables.

9

DESSERTS (CLEANSE)

Ah, the sweet taste of great health. Being on the candida diet doesn't mean going without, and these desserts will prove that to you. Treat yourself *and* enjoy your better health.

In this chapter:

Carob Clusters

Makes 6 Clusters

Fast, fast, fast! How long does it take to soothe your sweet tooth? Not long at all.

- ¼ cup coconut butter
- 1 tablespoon coconut oil
- 1 tablespoon carob powder or cacao powder
- 1 cup unsweetened shredded coconut
- ¼ cup ground flaxseed
- Pinch of stevia

1. In a double boiler or a bowl set atop a pot of gently simmering water, melt the coconut butter, oil, and carob powder. Once melted, add remaining ingredients to bowl and stir until combined.

2. If desired, top with seeds or nuts. Drop mixture into muffin cups. Stick in the freezer for 10 minutes, let sit for 20 minutes, and serve.

Nutty Seedy Truffles

Makes About 3 Dozen Truffles

Make a big batch of these and pop one if you get the urge. Reading the ingredient list you might think you're browsing in a health food store, but after tasting one truffle, you'll forget.

- 1 cup coconut milk
- 1 cup nut butter of your choice
- ½ cup chia seeds
- ½ cup coconut flour, divided
- ½ cup raw sesame seeds
- ½ cup raw hemp seeds
- ½ cup raw sunflower seeds
- Coconut shreds

1. In a blender, combine coconut milk, nut butter, and chia seeds. Blend until smooth and set aside.

2. In a large bowl, combine ¼ cup coconut flour, sesame seeds, hemp seeds, and sunflower seeds. Pour the blended mixture into the dry mixture.

3. Form a big ball with all the ingredients (except for the last ¼ cup coconut flour), and then create smaller truffle-sized balls of about 1 tablespoon of dough each.

4. Roll each ball in the remaining ¼ cup coconut flour, and then roll in coconut shreds.

Coconut Chocolate Brittle

Makes Almost 1 Full Pan

This delicious candy is easy to make and so good. The fact that it doesn't freeze entirely solid is actually great, because you can keep this in the freezer and eat it as you like.

- 1½ cups coconut oil
- 1 cup cacao powder
- 1 teaspoon vanilla extract (or to taste)

- 1 teaspoon stevia (or to taste)
- 30 raw almonds or hazelnuts

---

1. Melt coconut oil in a saucepan. Add cacao powder and stir until dissolved.

2. Add vanilla and stevia to taste a little at a time. If you add too much stevia, it will start to taste bitter.

3. Remove from heat and stir in nuts. Pour into a 9-by-13-inch pan lined with parchment paper. The paper should be long enough that you can pick up the edges once the brittle is finished.

4. Freeze the pan. Once the brittle is frozen, break into pieces. It won't be totally solid; use the parchment paper to lift out the brittle.

5. Store in the refrigerator or freezer.

Gingerbread Muffin Tops

Makes 8 Muffin Tops

Don't come unglued when you're trying to bake on the cleanse. When you're not using grains, you're gluten-free by definition, and gluten acts like glue—it makes everything stick together. Ground chia seeds, ground flaxseeds, or psyllium seed husks all work like magic in place of gluten. This recipe uses flaxseeds.

- ¼ cup coconut flour
- 1 tablespoon ground flaxseeds
- 1 tablespoon ground cinnamon
- 2 teaspoons ground ginger
- 1 teaspoon baking powder
- ⅛ teaspoon ground cloves
- ⅛ teaspoon grated nutmeg
- 1 cup egg whites (8 to 12, depending on the size of the eggs)
- ¼ cup coconut oil, melted
- ¼ cup canned coconut milk
- Liquid stevia to taste
- ½ teaspoon vanilla extract
- ¼ teaspoon almond extract

1. Preheat oven to 375°F and line a baking sheet with parchment paper.

2. Mix dry ingredients and set aside.

3. In a larger bowl, combine all wet ingredients with a hand mixer. Add dry to wet ingredients and mix until just combined.

4. Let the batter sit for several minutes to thicken. With a spoon, scoop the batter onto your prepared baking sheet, about 2 tablespoons' worth for each pile. Leave 1 inch between each stack.

5. If you do the stacks 1 tablespoon at a time, these are fluffier. In other words, first do a sheet with 1-tablespoon stacks; then go back and add another single tablespoon on top of each stack.

6. Bake for 18 to 20 minutes, or until a toothpick inserted into a muffin comes out clean and the edges are slightly golden.

7. You can also make mini muffins with the batter; bake at the same temperature, for 14 to 16 minutes. Regular- or larger-size muffins will not come out right.

No-Bake Coconut Chews

Makes 2 Dozen

This recipe really couldn't be much easier to make, and this sweet, chewy dessert is a real winner. (If you do make a mistake and end up with coconut butter, enjoy it.)

- 3 cups shredded unsweetened coconut
- 6 tablespoons coconut oil
- Stevia to taste
- 2 teaspoons vanilla extract
- ⅜ teaspoon sea salt

1. In a food processor or blender, combine all ingredients until the mixture is blended and sticks together. If you are using a high-powered blender like a Vitamix, do not turn your machine on high or you risk making coconut butter.

2. Form the mixture into desired shapes with your hands, a small cookie scoop, or a fruit baller.

No-Bake Coconut Almond Balls

Makes 3 Dozen

If you love nut butters, you won't be able to get enough of these. Another quick fix, too.

- ½ cup unsweetened shredded coconut, divided
- 1 cup almond butter or other nut butter
- ½ cup coconut flour
- 4 tablespoons coconut milk
- 4 tablespoons coconut oil
- Stevia to taste

1. Set aside a heaping tablespoon of the shredded coconut. Place all the other ingredients in a food processor or blender and blend until thoroughly combined.

2. Roll into bite-size balls and coat in remaining shredded coconut. Refrigerate for at least 30 minutes.

Lemon Pudding

Makes 1⅓ Cups

*This is a cool, delicious treat that will really shake up your menu. Don't skip
the refrigeration step.*

- 3 cups roughly chopped cauliflower
- 1 cup almond milk
- Stevia to taste

- 2 teaspoons vanilla extract
- Zest from 1 large lemon
- ¼ cup fresh lemon juice

---

1. Add cauliflower, almond milk, stevia, vanilla, and lemon zest to a
medium-sized saucepan. Bring to a boil on medium-high heat, uncovered.

2. Once it's boiling, reduce heat to a simmer and cook uncovered for 5
to 7 minutes, or until cauliflower is very soft. Remove from heat.

3. Place mixture in food processor or blender and add lemon juice.
Blend on high for 1 minute, or until very smooth.

4. Allow to cool uncovered at room temperature. Cover and refrigerate
for at least 18 hours.

PART 3
Recipes for Living Candida-Free

YOU'VE made it through the cleanse! At this stage your regimen gets much easier, and not just because your list of foods to enjoy grows. It's also because by now your symptoms have started to ease, your energy is increasing, and you're ready to take on more in general. Congratulations, you've earned some rewards!

NOW is not the time to go crazy, though. Remember that the way you got to this point was with hard work and determination. Your continued discipline will help transform what was an incredible challenge into a new way of life. Here is your transitional stage.

10

BREAKFAST (MAINTENANCE)

You've learned by now to power yourself up first thing, and now you've got more options than before! You can begin to slowly add in some fruits, too, which adds a new range of options for you.

In this chapter:

Buckwheat Sweet Potato Pancakes

Makes 8–10 pancakes

Sweet potatoes just for Thanksgiving? No way!

- 1 cup buckwheat flour
- ½ tablespoon baking powder
- ½ teaspoon ground cinnamon
- ½ teaspoon vanilla extract
- 1 egg
- ¼ cup mashed sweet potato
- 1 cup milk of your choice

---

1. In a large bowl, stir together buckwheat flour, baking powder, and cinnamon until blended. Add the vanilla, egg, sweet potato, and milk. Stir until just mixed.

2. Cook pancakes on lightly oiled nonstick pan. They're ready to turn when small bubbles form around the edges. Serve hot with butter and Sweet Almond Sauce (recipe on page 221).

Caramelized Onion "Quiche"

Makes 2 Servings

This is a hot, delicious breakfast that is perfect for a weekend get-together.

- 2 tablespoons coconut oil
- 1 large or two small yellow onions, thinly sliced
- 3 cloves garlic, minced
- 1 cup vegetable stock, divided
- ¼ cup finely ground flaxseeds
- 2 tablespoons finely ground chia seeds
- 1 tablespoon fresh lemon juice
- 1 tablespoon coconut aminos
- 5 drops stevia
- 1 cup raw natural almonds, finely ground
- ½ cup finely ground sunflower seeds
- ½ cup finely ground pumpkin seeds
- ¼ teaspoon sea salt
- ¼ teaspoon smoked paprika
- ¼ teaspoon baking soda
- ¼ teaspoon baking powder
- Black pepper to taste

---

1. Preheat oven to 350° F. Line a 9-by-9-inch square pan with parchment paper.

2. In a nonstick skillet, melt coconut oil over medium heat. Add onion and garlic and sauté until the onion begins to brown, 8–10 minutes, stirring frequently.

3. Add about half the vegetable stock, lower the heat, and cover the pan. Allow to cook until almost all the stock is absorbed and the onions are deep brown, about 20 minutes, stirring occasionally to prevent scorching. Turn off heat.

4. Add the remaining ingredients to the skillet and stir well to combine. Turn into the prepared pan; smooth the top. Bake 50 to 60 minutes, rotating the pan about halfway through, until the torte is slightly puffed and well browned. (Do not rely on the toothpick test; a tester may come out clean long before the torte is actually ready).

5. The torte will have a brown, slightly crisp exterior with a moist, grainy inside. It can be frozen.

Sweet Potato Hash Browns

Makes 2 Servings

Baking the sweet potato in advance (which you can do in the microwave) means that the cooking time is much shorter. It also means that the potato absorbs less fat, although it keeps all of its flavor.

- 1 tablespoon coconut oil
- 1 small yellow onion, diced
- ¼ to ½ pound meat, diced
- 2 cloves garlic, minced
- 2 cups cubed baked sweet potato
- Breakfast Seasoning (recipe on page 216)

---

1. Add coconut oil and diced onion to a large frying pan. Cook on medium-high heat for 5 minutes, stirring frequently.

2. Add meat and garlic and cook for 3 minutes, continuing to stir. Drop in cubed sweet potato and seasoning. Cook until as brown as you like.

Biscuits and Gravy

Makes 6 Biscuits

- 1 tablespoon fresh lemon juice, plus enough nut milk to equal 1 cup
- 1½ teaspoons vanilla extract
- 3 tablespoons finely ground flax seeds
- 10 drops stevia
- 2 tablespoons melted butter, plus 1 tablespoon for brushing tops

- ½ cup plus 1 tablespoon coconut flour
- 3 tablespoons buckwheat flour
- ¾ teaspoon baking powder
- ¾ teaspoon baking soda
- ¼ teaspoon sea salt
- Herb Gravy (recipe on page 109)

---

1. Preheat oven to 400°F. Line a cookie sheet with parchment paper.

2. Place the lemon juice in a measuring cup and add milk until the liquid measures 1 cup. In a bowl mix the lemon juice and milk mixture, vanilla, flax, stevia, and melted butter until evenly combined. Set aside for at least 2 minutes.

3. In a separate bowl, mix coconut flour, buckwheat flour, baking powder, baking soda, and sea salt. Combine wet and dry mixtures just to blend. Do not overmix. The mixture should be softer than a regular dough, yet still hold together, almost like a thick cookie dough.

4. Using a large scoop or ⅓-cup measuring cup, scoop the batter and place mounds on the cookie sheet. Flatten each mound slightly.

5. Bake for 12 minutes. Remove from the oven and brush gently with the remaining butter (the biscuits will be very delicate and can crush

easily). Rotate the pan and return to the oven for another 12 to 15 minutes, until tops are very deep golden brown. Do not underbake.

6. Remove from oven and cool on cookie sheet. These can be frozen.

7. If you try to eat these while they are still warm, the centers may seem too moist. Serve biscuits reheated and drenched in gravy.

Fried Eggs with Grilled Avocado and Coconut Bread

Makes 2 Servings

Take the first meal of the day as an opportunity to try something new and exciting. This dish featuring grilled avocado is the perfect chance.

- 1 large ripe avocado
- Squeeze of fresh lime juice
- Drizzle of olive oil
- 2 slices Coconut Bread (recipe on page 61), toasted, buttered if you like
- 2 eggs, fried
- Seasonings to taste

---

1. Heat indoor or outdoor grill. Sprinkle the cut surfaces of each avocado half with lime juice and olive oil.

2. Grill each side of avocado for about 2 minutes and serve on toast with fried eggs. Season to taste.

Green Machine Smoothie

Makes 1–2 Servings

Power yourself up with a smoothie that will invigorate you and keep you going all day.

- 1 cup Greek yogurt
- ½ medium lemon, peeled and deseeded
- ½ medium lime, peeled and deseeded
- Flesh of ½ ripe avocado
- 1 cup chopped greens (dandelion greens, kale, and/or spinach)
- Stevia to taste

Blend all ingredients on high until the smoothie is creamy.

Southwestern Omelet

Makes 1 Serving

Omelets are almost endlessly versatile. This one gives you a little kick for the rest of your day.

- ½ yellow onion, diced
- 1 clove garlic, minced
- 1 tablespoon olive oil
- ½ green bell pepper, diced
- ⅛ cup black beans, cooked
- ½ tomato, diced
- 2 eggs, beaten
- Guacamole for serving (recipe on page 62)

1. In a medium-sized skillet over medium-high heat, cook onion and garlic in olive oil until translucent.

2. Add bell pepper and cook until pepper is soft. Add beans and tomatoes to heat through.

3. Add eggs and cook until ready to turn. Flip omelet. Remove from pan and serve with guacamole.

Toad in the Hole

Makes 2 Servings

How about an old, comfortable favorite that's remade for your new lifestyle?

- 2 slices Coconut Bread (page 61) or Spinach Bread (page 138)
- Butter for cooking and serving
- 2 eggs

1. Tear holes in the middle of each slice of bread and butter the slices.

2. Over medium heat, melt generous amount of butter in medium-sized skillet. Place bread slices in skillet. Crack eggs with yolks intact into holes in bread. (According to your preference, you might want to break the yolks as they cook.)

3. Flip the slices and cook until the bread is golden-brown and the eggs are as done as you like.

11

SNACKS (MAINTENANCE)

Even though your meals might now be more filling, don't forget snacks. You definitely want to keep your body satisfied and put down any cravings that rear their ugly heads.

In this chapter:

Salsa

Corn-Free Chips

Spinach Bread

Syrian Red Pepper Dip

Quinoa Crackers

Almond Cheese

Salmon on Endive Spears

Deviled Eggs

Salsa

Makes About 2 Cups

Guess what you can eat a lot more of now? Tomatoes!

- 3 to 4 Roma tomatoes, chopped
- ½ red onion, minced
- ½ small cucumber, peeled, deseeded, and finely chopped
- ½ cup fresh cilantro, minced
- 1 clove garlic, minced
- Juice of 1 small lime
- Sea salt to taste

Combine all ingredients and chill to allow flavors to mingle.

Corn-Free Chips

Makes 6 Servings

Want to lay your hands on a crunchy, delicious snack? This is one of the best.

- ½ cup raw amaranth
- 1½ cups water
- ⅛ teaspoon sea salt
- Zest from 1 lime

1. Mix amaranth and water in a small, heavy saucepan. Cover and bring to a boil. Reduce heat to low and simmer for 20 to 25 minutes, or until all liquid is absorbed.

2. Remove from heat and transfer the cooked amaranth to a bowl. Allow the amaranth to chill for 30 minutes. Stir sea salt and lime zest into the cooled amaranth.

3. Preheat oven to 350°F and line a baking sheet with parchment paper.

4. Using a teaspoon, roll cooked amaranth into a ball. Press into a flattened circle about ⅛ inch thick on prepared baking sheet. The amaranth will be very sticky; just try your best to flatten and shape the chips until remaining amaranth is used up.

5. Bake for 15 minutes, rotate pan, and bake for another 10 minutes, or until crisp. Remove from the oven and allow to cool for 20 minutes. Store in an airtight container.

Spinach Bread

Makes 1 Loaf

This is one of the best breads for candida sufferers. It tastes great and it will work for anything from sandwiches to dips.

- 2½ cups almond flour
- ¼ teaspoon sea salt
- 2 teaspoons baking powder
- 1½ cups finely chopped or puréed fresh spinach
- 4 eggs, beaten
- ¼ cup coconut oil or olive oil, and for greasing pan
- 1 tablespoon apple cider vinegar or fresh lemon juice

---

1. Preheat oven to 350°F. In a large bowl, combine almond flour, sea salt, and baking powder.

2. Add spinach to other ingredients. Add the eggs, oil, and vinegar or lemon juice to mixture and combine thoroughly.

3. Scoop into a greased loaf pan and bake for 30 minutes, or until a toothpick inserted into the middle of the bread comes out clean. Cool and store in an airtight container or in the fridge or freezer.

Syrian Red Pepper Dip

Makes About 2 Cups

When health and convenience have to go hand in hand, there's no substitute for dipping. Cultures all over the world produce healthful, delicious dips. They're easy to make, simple to keep on hand, and wonderfully tasty. The next time you get a craving, take a dip.

- 3 red bell peppers
- 1 small red onion, chopped
- ¼ cup olive oil, divided
- ¾ cup walnuts
- 2 cloves garlic
- 1 tablespoon cayenne pepper
- ¼ teaspoon ground cumin
- Juice of ½ lemon
- Sea salt to taste

1. Roast red peppers using a gas stove or oven. For gas stoves, place the whole peppers directly on burners, flipping them with tongs until they are black all over. For ovens, roast the peppers for 10 to 12 minutes at 350°F on a baking tray covered with parchment paper, turning about every 4 minutes.

2. Peel off the skins from the peppers and remove the seeds and stem.

3. Sauté the onion in 1 tablespoon oil for 3 to 5 minutes.

4. Blend all ingredients in a food processor or blender until smooth.

5. Serve with Quinoa Crackers (recipe on page 140) or other crackers, chips, breads, or vegetables.

Quinoa Crackers

Makes 12 Servings

These crispy treats aren't just tasty and fun to eat. They're also a higher protein option than any other cracker.

- 1½ cups quinoa flour, plus extra for rolling out dough
- ¼ cup coconut oil
- ½ cup water
- 1 teaspoon baking soda
- ½ teaspoon sea salt
- ¼ teaspoon black pepper

1. Preheat the oven to 350°F. Lightly dust your work surface and a baking sheet with quinoa flour.

2. Combine all ingredients in a large bowl and mix thoroughly. Roll out dough on the floured work surface, turning the dough and sprinkling with additional flour as needed to prevent sticking.

3. When the dough is about ⅛ inch thick, cut it into shapes of your choice.

4. With a spatula, transfer the crackers to the baking sheet, prick each with a fork, and sprinkle with additional salt and pepper.

5. Bake for 20 minutes. Let the crackers cool for 1 hour before storing in an airtight container.

Almond Cheese

Makes About 1½ Cups

Are you missing cheese yet? Check this recipe out. You will love the flavor of this cheese, and it is far easier to make than you think.

- 1 cup raw almonds, soaked in water for 10 hours, then drained and blanched
- ¼ cup chopped fresh thyme leaves, plus extra for garnish
- ¼ cup water
- ¼ cup olive oil
- 2 cloves garlic
- ½ teaspoon sea salt
- Black pepper to taste

1. Combine all ingredients except for black pepper in a food processor. Process until the cheese has attained a smooth, creamy texture.

2. Season to taste with the pepper and additional salt. Place the cheese into a mold or bowl and chill until ready to serve.

3. Turn cheese out onto a serving plate and garnish with fresh thyme.

Salmon on Endive Spears

Makes 12 Spears

Entertaining while on this kind of regimen can be intimidating, but don't give up. There are options here that can please your guests, too, and this is one of the best.

- 1 (6 to 8-ounce) piece of salmon, cooked in olive oil in a skillet until just done, cooled, and flaked (this is a great vehicle for leftover salmon)
- ½ cup plain Greek yogurt
- 1 tablespoon fresh lemon juice
- 1 tablespoon chopped fresh tarragon
- Sea salt to taste
- 12 Belgian endive spears (about 2 heads)
- 1 tablespoon minced spring onion

1. In a bowl, mix salmon, yogurt, lemon, tarragon, and salt.

2. Scoop the mixture onto the endive spears. Garnish with spring onion and serve.

Deviled Eggs

Makes 4 Servings

This new take on an old favorite might taste even better than the original does. And if you really miss that mayonnaise flavor, you can make your own—check the recipe on page 211.

- 4 large eggs, hard boiled and cooled
- 3 tablespoons plain Greek yogurt
- 1 tablespoon fresh lemon juice
- ½ teaspoon dry mustard
- ½ teaspoon dried tarragon
- Paprika to taste and for garnish
- Sea salt and white pepper to taste
- 1 canned anchovy fillet

1. Peel shells from eggs, and then cut eggs in half. Take the yolks out of the eggs and mix in a bowl with the lemon juice and seasonings.

2. Place anchovy in bowl and mash with fork into paste. Add anchovy paste into yolk mixture to taste—be careful, it is strong.

3. Fill the hollowed-out egg whites with the yolk mixture and sprinkle a small amount of paprika over the top. Chill.

12

SOUPS, SALADS, SANDWICHES, AND SIDES (MAINTENANCE)

As the number of choices you have increases, so does your sense of freedom. Use the recipes in these chapters liberally, to keep variety in your menus.

In this chapter:

Zucchini Soup

Makes 2 Servings

This quick and easy soup makes use of one of the only squashes safe for all stages of the candida regimen.

- 2 zucchini, coarsely chopped
- 1 onion, coarsely chopped
- 2 cloves garlic
- 2 tablespoons olive oil
- Sea salt
- Water or milk of your choice

1. Steam the zucchini and onion until tender.

2. Purée the zucchini, onion, garlic, olive oil, and salt in your food processor or blender, adding only a small amount at a time. Add water or your preferred milk for desired consistency. Pour in bowls and serve.

Chunky Vegetable Soup

Makes 4–6 Servings

Supercharged with vegetable goodness, this soup is as satisfying as most more elaborate meals. This recipe makes a lot, so be ready to serve some friends or save the rest.

- 1 leek, sliced thin
- 1 yellow onion, diced
- 1 large stalk celery with green tops, sliced thin
- 4 cups chopped fresh green beans
- 6 cups chopped cabbage
- Vegetable stock or water to cover vegetables
- 1 cup chopped cauliflower florets
- 1 cup chopped broccoli florets
- 4 cloves garlic, minced
- ½ teaspoon dried thyme
- ½ teaspoon dried basil
- Sea salt and black pepper to taste
- Olive oil for serving

---

1. In a large stock pot cover leek, celery, onion, green beans, and cabbage with vegetable stock or water.

2. Bring to a boil, reduce heat to medium-low, cover pot, and simmer 10 minutes.

3. Add the rest of the ingredients except sea salt and olive oil, and add more liquid as necessary. Cover and simmer another 10 to 15 minutes.

4. Add sea salt and pepper to taste. Other seasonings such as dill and paprika are also great in this soup.

Chicken "Noodle" Soup

Makes About 1 Quart

You can add "noodles" to any soup using zucchini ribbons. Getting tired of those? You can eat soba noodles anytime, too.

- 1 quart chicken stock
- 1 rib celery, diced
- 1 large carrot, diced

- 1 small zucchini, made into noodles with a slicer or vegetable peeler

---

1. Bring chicken stock to a boil in a medium pot, and then reduce to a simmer.

2. Add celery and carrots to pot and simmer until tender, about 10 to 20 minutes. Add zucchini noodles and cook a few more minutes; do not overcook. Serve hot.

Cucumber, Dill, and Kale Salad

Makes 2 Servings

The tanginess of dill is a perfect fit for the cool crispiness of cucumber. Add to that the high-power nutrition of kale and onion, and your immune system will be thanking you all week.

- 2 bunches kale, torn into bite-sized pieces, thick stems discarded (about 4 cups)
- ½ cup cooked black beans
- Tangy Dill Dressing (recipe on page 210)
- ½ English cucumber, sliced with a vegetable peeler
- 1 whole carrot, diced
- 4 green onions, diced

---

1. Steam kale for 45 to 60 seconds, just to soften. Drain if needed and place in a large bowl.

2. Add remaining salad ingredients and stir to coat.

3. Store leftovers in the fridge in an airtight container for 1 to 2 days.

Taco Salad

Makes 2 Servings

This Southwestern treat is a meal more than a salad. Don't be intimidated by the ingredient list—this is easy.

- ½ white onion, sliced
- 3 tablespoons water
- 1 cup cooked chickpeas
- Chili powder, paprika, ground cumin, onion powder, dried oregano, garlic powder, red pepper flakes, sea salt, and black pepper to taste
- Guacamole (recipe on page 62)
- 2 cups chopped romaine lettuce
- 1 tomato, chopped
- 2 tablespoons Salsa (recipe on page 136)
- Corn-Free Chips (recipe on page 137)

1. To make the "meat," heat onion and water in a large saucepan over medium-high heat for 2 to 3 minutes until onion is softened. Add chickpeas and seasonings, and reduce heat to medium.

2. Cook uncovered for another 2 to 3 minutes, until heated through.

3. Meanwhile, combine lettuce, tomato, salsa, and chips in a bowl. Top salad with Guacamole and taco "meat" and serve.

Mock Caprese Salad

Makes 2 Servings

Do you have extra cheese around now that you've discovered how easy it is to make? Use it in this fantastic salad.

- 10 cherry tomatoes
- 10 pieces Almond Cheese (recipe on page 141)
- Handful of fresh basil leaves
- Olive oil
- Sea salt and black pepper to taste

1. Halve the cherry tomatoes and mix with the almond cheese and basil leaves.

2. Drizzle with olive oil and season with salt and pepper.

Pad Thai Salad

Makes 2 Servings

Although traditional Thai food makes heavy use of peanuts, which are forbidden on the candida diet, you'll be thrilled with the way sunflower butter works here. Grating or spiralizing (with a tool called a spiralizer) work equally well for the vegetables.

For the salad:

- 1 large zucchini, spiralized or grated
- 1 small carrot, spiralized or grated
- Handful of bean sprouts
- 1 cup thinly sliced purple cabbage
- 3 green onions, chopped
- 2 tablespoons chopped fresh cilantro
- Juice of ½ lime

For the dressing:

- 1 teaspoon sunflower seed butter
- 1 teaspoon water
- 1 tablespoon fresh lime juice
- ½ teaspoon coconut aminos
- 2 tablespoons chopped fresh cilantro
- ¼ small jalapeño, chopped
- 1 clove garlic, minced

1. Combine all salad ingredients in a large bowl.

2. Blend all dressing ingredients in a food processor or blender until smooth, about 30 seconds. Pour the dressing over the salad, stir to coat, and serve.

Mediterranean Chickpea Patties

Makes 8 Patties

These patties are awesome on bread or on their own. You can even top them with homemade cheese and homemade condiments.

- 1 pound cooked chickpeas
- ½ cup chopped fresh flat-leaf parsley
- 3 cloves garlic, chopped, or adjust this to taste
- ¼ teaspoon ground cumin
- 1 teaspoon sea salt, divided
- 1 teaspoon black pepper, divided
- 1 egg, beaten
- 4 tablespoons flour of your choice, divided
- 2 tablespoons olive oil

1. In a food processor, pulse first four ingredients and ½ teaspoon each of the sea salt and black pepper until coarsely chopped.

2. Once the patty mixture comes together, transfer it to a mixing bowl and add egg and 2 tablespoons flour.

3. Form 8 patties out of this mixture. They should be about ½ inch thick. Put the remaining flour into a shallow dish and roll the patties in it. Tap excess flour off the patties.

4. In a wide, nonstick skillet, heat olive oil over medium-high heat. Cook patties for 2 to 3 minutes on each side, or until golden brown.

5. Serve on any candida-safe bread or a candida-safe wrap. Try with Macadamia Nut "Hummus" (recipe on page 63) or any of the delicious sauces and dressings in Chapter 16.

Mashed Notatoes

Makes 4 Servings

This is another side dish that will show you that living candida-free doesn't mean going without the foods you love to eat. Butter is one of the only dairy products that is green-lighted on your regimen.

- 2 heads cauliflower, washed and cut into large pieces
- 2 tablespoons butter (or more to taste)

- 2 tablespoons Greek yogurt
- Sea salt to taste
- Additional butter and Greek yogurt for serving, if desired

1. Steam the cauliflower pieces until very tender.

2. Purée cauliflower in a food processor, add all other ingredients, and continue to blend until smooth.

3. Reheat in a casserole dish in the oven at 350°F for 20 minutes and serve. Serve with additional butter and yogurt if desired.

Broccoli Rabe and Garlic

Makes 2 Servings

This vegetable is a wonderful green option that you don't see every day. You're going to love the delicate flavor, and your digestive system will love how you're treating it.

- 1 bunch broccoli rabe, tough stems on bottom trimmed off and discarded
- 2 tablespoons olive oil
- 10 cloves garlic, left whole
- ¼ teaspoon sea salt
- ¼ teaspoon black pepper

1. In a large skillet heat oil. Add garlic to skillet and cook over medium heat until lightly browned, a few minutes.

2. Add broccoli rabe to skillet and cook until just wilted. Sprinkle with salt and pepper and serve.

Eggplant Caponata

Makes 2 Servings

Such a delicious, easy dish. You will adore the flavor.

- 1 medium eggplant, skin on, diced into ½-inch cubes
- 1 stalk celery, diced
- ½ cup cherry tomatoes, sliced in half
- 2 tablespoons kalamata olives, sliced in half
- 1/2 small yellow onion, diced
- 2 to 4 tablespoons olive oil
- ¼ teaspoon sea salt

1. Preheat oven to 350°F. Combine all ingredients in a 9-by-13-inch oven-proof baking dish.

2. Bake for 35 to 45 minutes, or until eggplant is tender, and serve.

Grilled Zucchini

Makes 2 Servings

This simple, tasty side dish will complement almost any main dish. The grilled flavor is a special treat.

- 3 to 4 small zucchini
- 2 tablespoons olive oil

- 1 teaspoon sea salt

---

1. Trim off the ends of the zucchini; then cut each zucchini in half. Cut each half lengthwise into ½-inch-thick strips.

2. In a large bowl, toss zucchini with olive oil and salt.

3. Grill zucchini on each side for 3 to 6 minutes, until zucchini is tender and has grill marks on each side. Serve hot.

13

MAIN DISHES (MAINTENANCE)

R eady to hear about more amazing meals you can treat yourself to while boosting your health and extending your life? These main dishes are going to seem more decadent than the last batch, mostly because as you move toward maintaining your new candida-free lifestyle, you're more able to accommodate legumes, tomatoes, certain fruits, and other foods you've been missing.

In this chapter:

Mediterranean Stew

Makes 4–6 Servings

This stew is a stew in name only; it is absolutely a meal. The kasha especially lends it substance, and the spices and olives provide unbeatable flavor.

- 2 red bell peppers
- 1 tablespoon olive oil
- 1 large yellow onion, diced
- 2 shallots, finely chopped
- 3 cloves garlic, minced
- 6 cups vegetable stock
- 1 (28-ounce) can whole tomatoes, drained
- 1½ cups raw buckwheat groats, rinsed
- 2 tablespoons apple cider vinegar
- 2 sprigs fresh rosemary
- ½ teaspoon dried marjoram
- 2 cups chopped eggplant
- 1 cup baby spinach
- ½ cup pitted and sliced black olives
- ½ teaspoon sea salt
- Black pepper to taste

---

1. Roast bell peppers using a gas stove or oven. For a gas stove, place the whole peppers directly on the burners, flipping them with tongs until they are black all over. For an oven, roast the peppers for 10 to 12 minutes at 350°F on a baking tray covered with parchment paper, turning about every 4 minutes. Peel off the skins from the peppers and remove the seeds and stems. Cut into strips.

2. Heat oil in a large saucepan on medium-high heat. Add onion, shallots, and garlic and sauté until soft and translucent, about 10 minutes.

3. Add stock, tomatoes, buckwheat, vinegar, rosemary, and marjoram. Cover, bring to a boil, and reduce heat to low. Simmer until the buckwheat is tender, about 20 to 25 minutes.

4. Stir in the chopped eggplant about 10 minutes into the simmering time.

5. Once the buckwheat is tender, stir in the roasted red peppers, spinach, and olives. Cook just until the peppers and olives are heated through and spinach is wilted.

6. Season with salt and pepper. Remove rosemary sprigs before serving.

Coconut Lamb Curry

Makes 4 Servings

If you haven't tried lamb, you really should. It's tender and rich, and just as easy to cook with as anything else.

- 1 medium onion, chopped
- 2 cloves garlic, minced
- 1 mild to medium chile, seeds discarded, chopped
- 1 tablespoon coconut oil
- 1 pound boneless lamb, cubed
- 4 medium tomatoes, chopped
- 1 can coconut milk
- ½ teaspoon cayenne pepper
- ½ teaspoon ground turmeric
- ½ teaspoon curry powder or garam masala
- Sea salt to taste

1. In a broad, deep saucepan, cook onion, garlic, and chile in coconut oil until onion and garlic are translucent.

2. Add lamb and cook over medium heat for 5 minutes.

3. Add all the other ingredients and simmer for 30 minutes more over low heat.

4. Serve with a small portion of wild or brown rice.

Slow-Cooker Chicken

Makes 4–6 Servings

Take advantage of your slow cooker. Just pop everything in and forget about it until later.

- 1 sweet potato or other root vegetable, cubed
- ½ pound green beans, ends snapped off, cut into bite-size pieces
- 1 onion, chopped
- 1 celery stalk, chopped
- 1 bulb fennel, chopped into small pieces
- 4 chicken breasts, cubed
- 3 to 5 cloves garlic
- Garlic powder, salt, black pepper, paprika, and other seasonings that work with the meat you choose, to taste (herbes de Provence are another good choice for chicken)
- Chicken stock, homemade or canned, that passes the candida label test

Place all ingredients in slow cooker and cook on high for 5 hours or low for 7 to 8 hours.

Grilled Lemon Chicken

Makes 4 Servings

Something this simple can be completely delicious. You'll master the recipe in no time.

- ⅓ cup fresh lemon juice
- ⅓ cup olive oil
- 1 teaspoon sea salt
- ½ teaspoon black pepper
- 1½ teaspoons minced fresh thyme leaves

- 1 pound boneless, skinless chicken breasts, halved
- 1 head romaine lettuce
- 2 large carrots, grated or julienned
- Any sauce or dressing from this book of your choice

---

1. In a medium bowl, whisk together lemon juice, olive oil, salt, pepper, and thyme to make the marinade.

2. Place chicken and marinade in a resealable plastic bag and marinate overnight.

3. When ready to cook, grill chicken for 10 minutes on each side, or until cooked through. Cool chicken and cut diagonally into ½-inch-thick slices.

4. Remove bottoms of romaine lettuce and cut leaves into long, thin strips. Place romaine on a serving platter and top with grated or julienned carrots.

5. Place chicken over vegetables and serve with candida-safe sauce or dressing of your choice.

Vegetarian Nasi Goreng

Makes 2 Servings

Cook things like quinoa in large amounts on the weekend when you have time. It makes it easy if you have it on hand during the week. It's perfect with this recipe, which you shouldn't be afraid of trying despite the exotic name.

- 2 eggs
- 2 red onions, one coarsely chopped, the other thinly sliced
- 2 red chiles, 1½ of them thinly sliced (don't worry about seeds)
- 3 cloves garlic, peeled
- 4 tablespoons sesame oil
- 1 yellow bell pepper, thinly sliced
- 1 carrot, sliced with a peeler
- 2 cups cooked kasha, quinoa, diced steamed cauliflower, or any other rice replacement*
- 2 spring onions, cut lengthwise
- Handful of cilantro, chopped
- Sea salt to taste

1. Scramble the eggs in a large, deep skillet and set them aside.

2. In a food processor or blender, mix the chopped red onion, the half red chile, and the garlic at high speed to make a paste.

3. Add the sesame oil and the paste to your skillet and cook at medium high heat for 3 minutes.

4. Reduce heat to medium and add the remaining sliced red onion, sliced red chiles, yellow bell pepper, and carrot, and cook for about 2 minutes.

5. Add the rice replacement and cook for another 2 minutes.

6. Finally, mix in the eggs, spring onion, and cilantro and cook for 1 minute. Serve hot.

*If you're in the maintenance stage, you may use wild rice.

Lamb Pasticcio

Makes 4 Servings

The hardest part about making this dish is waiting for it to come out of the oven while you smell it cooking. The word pasticcio *means "hodgepodge" or "mess" in Italian, but that term is an affectionate one.*

- Olive oil
- 1 large onion, chopped
- 2 cloves garlic, minced
- 1 pound boneless lamb meat, minced
- 2 cups baby spinach, chopped
- ¾ cup vegetable stock
- Sea salt and black pepper to taste
- 1½ teaspoons ground cinnamon
- 4 ounces dry buckwheat pasta, preferably smaller pasta
- 1 tablespoon buckwheat flour
- 2 medium tomatoes, sliced
- 2 eggs, beaten
- 1½ cups plain Greek yogurt

1. Preheat oven to 375°F. Heat the oil in a large, deep-lidded skillet big enough to accommodate all ingredients.

2. Add onion and garlic and cook over medium-high heat until soft and translucent.

3. Add the lamb and spinach and cook until the lamb browns. Add the stock, salt, pepper, and cinnamon. Bring to a boil, cover, and let simmer for 15 minutes.

4. Stir the dry pasta and flour into the mixture. Spoon into a deep 13-by-9-inch ovenproof dish and place tomato slices on top.

5. In a separate bowl, beat the eggs together with the yogurt, and then spread evenly over the mixture. Bake for 45 minutes, and then serve.

Veggie Burgers

Makes 4 Servings

These veggie burgers are full of protein and great flavor. These are far better than you think and even have a delicious, crisp texture on the outside.

- 1 pound cooked chickpeas
- 2 cups fresh spinach
- ¼ cup chopped red onion
- 1/3 cup ground flaxseeds
- 1 teaspoon sea salt
- 1 teaspoon black pepper
- ½ tablespoon garlic powder
- 1 teaspoon dried dill

1. Place all ingredients in a food processor or blender. Slowly combine, increasing speed gradually as mixture begins to resemble cookie dough. Form into 4 burger patties.

2. Heat grill or turn stove on to medium-high. Cook burgers on each side for 7 to 8 minutes. They should be lightly brown and soft like a hamburger, but crunchy on the outside.

3. Serve on bread or with condiments or cheese from this book's recipes, or topped with grilled or raw veggies.

Spaghetti Squash and Meatballs

Makes 4 Servings

Heads up for some more comfort food. These amazing meatballs dress up the spaghetti squash—one of nature's most amazing creations.

For the spaghetti squash:
- 1 large spaghetti squash
- 4 to 6 teaspoons coconut oil
- Dried rosemary, dried thyme, sea salt, black pepper, or other seasonings to taste

For the meatballs:
- 1 large onion, chopped
- 2 cloves garlic, minced
- 2 tablespoons olive oil
- 1 egg, beaten
- 1 pound turkey or chicken breasts or beef, minced (mince them yourself)
- 2 pieces Basic Candida-Safe Bread (recipe on page 222)
- Sea salt and black pepper to taste
- 1 tablespoon ground flaxseeds
- ¼ cup fresh parsley, minced
- Homemade stock of your choice for cooking meatballs (you can supplement with water)
- Oil for greasing baking sheet

For the sauce:
- 4 Roma tomatoes, chopped
- Dried oregano, basil, garlic powder, sea salt, black pepper, or other seasonings to taste

---

1. Preheat oven to 350° F. Slice squash in half. Dig out seeds. Put 2–3 teaspoons coconut oil in each squash half. Season each half to taste and turn them cut side down in a well-oiled pan.

2. Bake the squash for about 1 hour, or until tender.

2. Meanwhile, make the meatballs. In a large skillet over medium-high heat, brown onion and garlic in olive oil. Set aside to cool slightly. Save the skillet for the tomatoes.

3. In a bowl, mix egg, minced meat, onions, and garlic. Toast bread and crumble with your hands into bread crumbs. Add crumbs, salt, pepper, flaxseeds, and parsley to the bowl. Season as you see fit. Shape into meatballs.

4. Bring stock (and extra water for volume if needed) to boil in a pot big enough to accommodate the meatballs. Simmer meatballs for 10 minutes.

5. Remove meatballs from the stock with a slotted spoon and place on an oiled baking sheet. Ensure oil covers surfaces of the meatballs.

6. When the squash is done, bake the meatballs for 15 to 25 minutes, depending on the size of the balls. This allows them to cook through and brown. You can put them in the oven alongside the squash, but this may extend the cooking time for both.

7. In the skillet with the oil and onion and garlic drippings, briefly heat the chopped tomatoes and season them to taste to make your sauce.

8. When squash is finished, use a fork to pull the squash out in strands. Put this "spaghetti" on a plate. Add tomatoes and meatballs and serve.

Chicken Parmesan

Makes 2 Servings

It's true that without actual Parmesan, this dish is an imposter. But you won't care the moment you try it.

- 4 slices Basic Candida-Safe Bread (recipe on page 222) for crumb mixture
- ½ teaspoon each onion powder, dried parsley, dried oregano, black pepper, and sea salt
- 1 egg, beaten
- Small amount of milk of your choice for coating meat
- Olive oil for frying
- 2 boneless, skinless chicken breasts
- 2 thin slices Almond Cheese (recipe on page 141)
- 1 tomato, sliced

1. Toast bread slices and crumble with your hands. Add seasonings and mix. Place in a wide, shallow bowl.

2. Mix egg and milk in a smaller, shallow bowl.

3. In a large, deep skillet, place olive oil for frying on medium to medium-high heat. The oil is hot enough when crumbs tossed in pan sizzle; it is too hot if it smokes or spits.

4. Coat each breast in the egg-milk mixture and then coat well in crumbs. Put into hot skillet. Lower heat slightly and cook coated breasts, uncovered, until done through. Check with a thermometer or by slicing through thickest parts.

5. Top each cooked breast while still very hot with a slice of cheese and a slice of tomato.

Zucchini Casserole

Makes 8 Servings

What will likely surprise you most about this dish is its richness. You can also add candida-safe bread crumbs and/or cheese.

- 1 cup cooked quinoa
- 2 to 3 cups thinly sliced zucchini
- ½ cup chopped green onions
- ¼ cup chopped fresh parsley
- ¼ cup olive oil
- 2 to 3 eggs, beaten
- ½ teaspoon sea salt
- ¼ teaspoon garlic powder
- ½ teaspoon dried oregano

Preheat oven to 350°F. Combine all ingredients thoroughly in an oiled 8-by-8-inch casserole dish. Bake for 45 minutes to 1 hour, or until eggs are set.

Garlic-Braised Eggplant and Chickpea Casserole

Makes 4 Servings

Always cook beans yourself unless you absolutely can't. When you do, cook them in homemade veggie or chicken stock instead of water and you will be amazed at how much more delicious they taste. Use water if you're making something sweet with them.

- ¼ cup plus 2 tablespoons olive oil
- 1½ teaspoons cumin seeds
- ½ teaspoon fennel seeds
- ½ teaspoon cracked peppercorns
- 2 medium-sized yellow onions, thinly sliced
- 12 large cloves garlic, thinly sliced
- 2 teaspoons mustard powder
- 1 teaspoon red pepper flakes
- 1 teaspoon ground turmeric
- 1 teaspoon sea salt
- 1 small eggplant, unpeeled, cut into pieces about ½ inch thick and 2 inches long
- 5 plum tomatoes, quartered lengthwise
- 2½ cups cooked chickpeas
- 2 tablespoons chopped fresh cilantro

1. In large, deep skillet, heat the oil, add cumin seeds, and cook until brown, about 15 seconds. Add the fennel seeds and cracked peppercorns and cook for 5 seconds more.

2. Add the onions and garlic and reduce heat to medium-high. Cook, stirring often, until the onions and garlic are lightly browned.

3. Stir in the mustard, pepper flakes, turmeric, and salt. Add the eggplant. Reduce the heat to medium and cook, stirring gently until eggplant is soft, about 5 minutes.

4. Add the tomatoes and cook, stirring constantly, about 5 minutes more, or until tomatoes are soft.

5. Gently stir in chickpeas. Cover and simmer over low heat until liquid thickens to gravy. Season with additional salt to taste. Sprinkle with cilantro and serve.

Simple Southwestern Quinoa and Beans

Makes 1 Serving

Rice and beans are a staple dish around the world for good reason. With quinoa standing in for rice, you're not only candida-safe, you're even higher in protein.

- ½ yellow onion, diced
- 1 clove garlic, minced
- 2 tablespoons olive oil
- 1 cup cooked quinoa
- ½ cup cooked black beans
- Ground cumin, dried oregano, chili powder, cayenne, sea salt, and black pepper to taste
- Several leaves romaine lettuce, chopped
- 1 small tomato, chopped
- Greek yogurt
- Corn-Free Chips (recipe on page 137) or Buckwheat Tortillas (recipe on page 223)

---

1. In a large, deep skillet, cook onion and garlic in olive oil until translucent.

2. Add quinoa, black beans, and seasonings to taste. Heat through. Serve immediately with chopped lettuce, tomato, yogurt, and chips or tortillas.

Salmon Lettuce Wraps

Makes 2 Servings

Lettuce wraps are tasty and fun. Try them with other meats, or even chickpeas, once you are in the maintenance phase.

- 1 red onion, diced
- 1 jalapeño, diced
- 1 tablespoon coconut oil
- 2 salmon fillets (about ¼–½ pound)
- Dash of cayenne
- Salt to taste

- 5 or 6 large romaine or butter lettuce leaves
- Salsa (recipe on page 136) or other dip
- 1 small cucumber, chopped
- Two limes, quartered

---

1. In a large skillet, sauté onion and jalapeño in coconut oil over medium-high heat until onions are translucent.

2. Season salmon with salt and cayenne and add to skillet. Cook for about 4 to 5 minutes on each side, until middle is opaque but not overdone. Set aside to cool.

3. Chop salmon into large chunks. Top lettuce leaves with fish, salsa, and cucumber. Squeeze lime juice over each wrap and serve.

Beef Fajitas

Makes 4 Servings

It is easy to get the knack of this traditional method for making fajitas, and well worth the effort. Serve them sizzling hot.

- Juice of 1 lime
- 3 tablespoons olive oil, divided
- 2 cloves garlic, peeled and minced
- ½ teaspoon ground cumin
- ½ fresh jalapeño pepper, seeded, ribs removed, and finely chopped
- ¼ cup chopped fresh cilantro
- 1 pound flank steak or skirt steak
- 1 large yellow onion, peeled

- 2 or 3 bell peppers of various colors, stemmed, seeded, de-ribbed, and sliced lengthwise into strips
- Sea salt to taste
- Salsa (recipe on page 136)
- Guacamole (recipe on page 62)
- Kale (steamed for 1 minute and chopped) or romaine lettuce (chopped)
- Greek yogurt
- Buckwheat Tortillas (recipe on page 223)

1. Combine lime juice, 2 tablespoons olive oil, garlic, cumin, jalapeño, and cilantro to make marinade. Coat steak with marinade and let sit at room temperature for an hour or longer if refrigerated.

2. While steak is marinating, slice onion. Prepare the bell peppers.

3. Set a large cast iron pan or griddle over high heat and let it heat up for 1 to 2 minutes. Add 1 tablespoon oil to the pan and let it heat up for 1 minute.

4. Wipe off most of the marinade from the steak and salt it. Add to the hot pan, frying each side for 3 minutes, or to desired doneness; 3 minutes per side will yield medium-rare doneness for an average cut of flank steak. Skirt steak needs less time. If the pan starts to smoke too much, reduce the heat to medium-high. Avoid burning.

5. After cooking, remove the steak from the pan and let it sit, tented with foil, for 5 minutes.

6. While meat is resting, add a little more oil to the pan if necessary, and then add the onions and bell peppers. Let these sear for 1 minute before stirring; then stir every 90 seconds or so as the veggies sear. Cook for 5 to 6 minutes total.

7. After it has rested, slice the steak against the grain into thin slices. If you slice the meat at an angle, you will be able to get your slices pretty thin. These cuts of steak are flavorful but can be a little tough, so thin slices will help make them easier to eat.

8. Serve immediately with salsa, guacamole, chopped kale or romaine lettuce, Greek yogurt, and warm buckwheat tortillas.

Vegetable Fritters

Makes 10 Fritters

These fritters are tasty and addictive. If you haven't had fritters that aren't sweet, you are in for a treat with these.

- 3 zucchini, grated
- Pinch of salt
- ¼ cup finely chopped cauliflower
- 1 cup finely chopped fresh spinach
- ½ onion, finely chopped
- 1 clove garlic, crushed
- 1 tablespoon chopped fresh parsley
- 1 tablespoon chopped fresh mint
- Sea salt and black pepper to taste
- Zest from 1 lemon
- 3 eggs, lightly beaten
- ½ cup almond meal
- 1 tablespoon coconut oil

---

1. Place zucchini into a colander and sprinkle it with a pinch of salt. Let sit for about 10 minutes to "sweat." Squeeze as much excess moisture from the zucchini as possible and place in a mixing bowl.

2. Add remaining ingredients and mix well; mixture should hold together nicely.

3. Place a large, deep skillet over medium heat and add coconut oil. Cook fritters for 3 minutes on each side, or until golden. Transfer them to a plate to keep warm as the others cook.

Zucchini, Celery, and Nut Loaf

Makes 1 Loaf

If you think this sounds too "veggie" for you, think again. This holds together beautifully, and you'll be more than happy to eat the leftovers.

- 4 tablespoons olive oil, divided, and to oil pan
- 1 onion, diced
- 2 cloves garlic, crushed
- 2 celery sticks, diced
- Seasoning to taste
- 1½ cups almond meal
- ½ teaspoon stevia powder
- ½ teaspoon sea salt
- ½ teaspoon baking powder
- 1 egg, lightly beaten
- 2 tablespoons almond milk
- 3 zucchini, grated and drained
- 1½ cups chopped mixed raw walnuts and Brazil nuts
- 1 tablespoon grated lemon zest

1. Preheat the oven to 350°F and oil a standard-size loaf pan.

2. Heat half the oil in a large, deep pan over medium heat. Add the onion, garlic, celery, and herbs and cook, stirring often, until the onion is translucent. Set aside.

3. In a large bowl, combine the almond flour, stevia, salt, and baking powder.

4. Add the egg, the remaining oil, the almond milk, zucchini, walnuts, Brazil nuts, and lemon zest and mix well.

5. Pour into the prepared pan and bake for 30 to 40 minutes, or until crispy and brown on top and set in the middle.

6. Cool for 10 minutes in the pan to allow the loaf to firm up, and then turn out onto a rack to cool completely.

7. Cut into slices to serve. The loaf will keep well for 4 days in the fridge in a well-sealed container or firmly wrapped in foil.

14

DESSERTS (MAINTENANCE)

Just like the main dishes in Chapter 13, these desserts are more decadent and satisfying thanks to the presence of fruit and other ingredients you might have been missing. As you near the end of this book, you can see how easy a successful anti-candida regimen really is. Living candida-free over the long term is completely possible.

Every time baking soda and baking powder are referred to in this book, as with everything else, it is the gluten-free versions that are needed. You'll also want to buy vanilla extract without alcohol.

In this chapter:

Strawberries and Crushed Walnuts
Yogurt and Frozen Raspberries
Yogurt Pudding

Carob Fudge
Rhubarb Pie
Sweet Zucchini Muffins
Vanilla Frosted Cupcakes
Sea Salt Brownies

Strawberries and Crushed Walnuts

Makes 1 Serving

Want to satisfy your sweet tooth without spending hours in the kitchen? Check out these quick and easy treats.

- 5 to 6 fresh strawberries
- ¼ cup crushed walnuts
- Sweet Almond Sauce (recipe on page 221)

---

1. Slice the strawberries and sprinkle with crushed walnuts. Drizzle with Sweet Almond Sauce.

2. As a variation, you can modify Sweet Almond Sauce by making it with walnuts.

Yogurt and Frozen Raspberries

Makes 1 Serving

Not used to your desserts being packed with protein and antioxidants? Get used to it.

- ¼ cup frozen raspberries
- ½ cup Greek yogurt
- Stevia to taste
- Crushed nuts (optional)

Mash frozen fruit in a bowl. Add yogurt, stevia, and nuts and stir. Now it's ready to eat.

Yogurt Pudding

Makes 1 Serving

Think of this recipe as a versatile starting point. You can use any nut butter you like, then add unsweetened cacao and any allowable add-ins on your list. Make it your own.

- ½ cup Greek yogurt
- 2 tablespoons nut butter
- Stevia to taste
- Ground cinnamon to taste

Mix all ingredients in a bowl. Serve at once or after chilling in freezer for 10 minutes for a cold treat.

Carob Fudge

Makes 2 Cups Fudge

The only thing better than the easiness of this recipe is how rich and delectable a confection it makes.

- 2 cups hazelnut or other nut butter
- 4 tablespoons unsweetened carob powder

Blend ingredients. Spread in small oiled pan and freeze for at least 1 hour to achieve a fudge-like consistency.

Rhubarb Pie

Makes 1 Pie

Ready to flex your muscles and impress your friends? Not to mention making your neighbors jealous—wait until you smell your kitchen when you bake up this gorgeous pie.

For the crust:

- 2¼ cups almond flour
- 1 teaspoon sea salt
- 2 packets stevia
- 1 stick (½ cup) salted butter, at room temperature
- ½ teaspoon vanilla extract

For the filling:

- 5 cups 1-inch slices fresh rhubarb
- 1 tablespoon fresh lemon juice
- 1 teaspoon vanilla extract
- 1 teaspoon stevia (or more, to taste)
- ¼ teaspoon grated nutmeg
- ½ teaspoon ground cinnamon
- 1 tablespoon chia seeds
- ¼ teaspoon salt
- 2 tablespoons salted butter
- 1 tablespoon coconut flour

1. Preheat oven to 350°F. To make the crust, combine the almond flour, salt, and stevia in a large bowl and mix them together thoroughly.

2. Add the butter and vanilla and stir until all ingredients are evenly incorporated. Transfer the piecrust dough to a pie pan. Use your hands to gently push the dough across the bottom of the pan and up the sides until it reaches the desired height. The crust should be about ¼ inch thick. You can prebake the crust for 5 to 10 minutes at 350°F to accentuate a toasted, brown-butter flavor in the almond flour.

(If you are an experienced baker, you may have noticed that a properly made pie crust demands ice-cold butter and a pastry cutter or a food processor. However, given that this is a specialized recipe with more delicate ingredients, it is important to keep the crust together. This is why the butter must be soft. Do not be concerned about this.)

3. In a large bowl, combine the rhubarb with lemon juice, vanilla, stevia, nutmeg, cinnamon, chia seeds, and salt. Toss the fruit lightly, either with your hands or using a kitchen utensil and a gentle folding motion to coat the rhubarb with the ingredients.

4. In a large pan over medium heat, melt the salted butter. To the melted butter, add the coated fruit and coconut flour.

5. Over medium to low heat, cook this mixture on the stove top for 5 minutes to soften the rhubarb and allow the pie filling to thicken.

6. Pour the rhubarb mixture into the prebaked pie shell. In order to avoid burning the edges of the pie's crust, cover the exposed crust with tinfoil. Bake the pie for 40 minutes.

Sweet Zucchini Muffins

Makes 12 Muffins

- 1½ cups almond flour
- 1 cup coconut flour
- ½ cup hazelnut flour
- ½ teaspoon salt
- 1 teaspoon grated nutmeg
- 3 teaspoons ground cinnamon
- ¼ teaspoon baking soda
- 4 eggs, beaten
- ½ cup milk of your choice
- 12 tablespoons (1½ sticks) salted butter, at room temperature
- 2 tablespoons Greek yogurt
- 2 teaspoons vanilla extract
- 2 teaspoons liquid stevia
- 2 teaspoons fresh lemon juice
- 1 teaspoon lemon zest
- 4 cups finely grated zucchini
- ½ cup chopped walnuts

---

1. Preheat oven to 350° F. In a large bowl, combine the almond, coconut, and hazelnut flours.

2. Add the salt, nutmeg, cinnamon, and baking soda. Set aside.

3. Mix all wet ingredients except zucchini in a different bowl until combined. Add the finely shredded zucchini to the wet mixture and stir a few times to coat the zucchini.

4. Add the wet ingredients to the dry ingredients and stir to thoroughly combine into a thick, sticky batter.

5. Add the chopped walnuts and fold them evenly into the batter.

6. Scoop the muffins into a cup-lined muffin tray, using your hands to shape the batter in the cups.

7. Bake the muffins for 30 minutes, or until the tops appear golden brown at the edges. Serve plain or toasted and buttered.

8. Keep these muffins in the refrigerator or store in the freezer and defrost as needed.

Vanilla Frosted Cupcakes

Makes 12 Cupcakes

Ground nuts are a wonderful substitute for grain flours, and as long as you avoid peanuts, cashews, and pistachios, you're home free, even in the cleanse stage. Grinding nuts finely until they resemble breadcrumbs or powder is one of the best ways to replace traditional flour in baking. Just don't grind too long or you'll have delicious homemade nut butter instead.

For the vanilla buttercream:
- 2 cans unsweetened coconut milk, refrigerated for at least 1 hour
- 1 stick (½ cup) salted butter, at room temperature
- 1 teaspoon vanilla extract
- 2 teaspoons liquid stevia

For the cupcakes:
- 1 (15-ounce) can organic butter beans (in water, with no added ingredients)
- ½ cup unsweetened liquid coconut milk (retained from icing)
- 2 eggs, beaten
- 1¾ teaspoon liquid stevia
- 2 teaspoon vanilla extract
- 4 tablespoons salted butter, melted
- 1½ cups almond flour
- ½ teaspoon salt
- ¼ teaspoon baking soda
- ⅛ teaspoon cream of tartar
- ¼ teaspoon fresh lemon juice

1. To make the frosting, separate the fat from the cold cans of unsweetened coconut milk by skimming off the milk solids from the top of the liquid. Save the liquid for the cupcakes.

2. Place the milk solids, butter, vanilla, and stevia in a food processor or blender and pulse until just blended. Small lumps are fine; do not over-process or your butter will separate, which will ruin the icing.

3. Preheat the oven to 350°F. To make the cupcakes, strain and rinse the butter beans to wash off excess starches. Rinse until the water runs clear out of the strainer.

4. In the bowl of a food processor, combine the beans, coconut liquid, eggs, stevia, vanilla, and melted butter. Purée these until they come together in a smooth, paste-like batter. No beans should be left whole.

5. To the puréed wet ingredients, add the almond flour, salt, baking soda, cream of tartar, and lemon juice. Run the food processor again to integrate all the ingredients.

6. Line a cupcake pan with liners. Fill each liner three-fourths full.

7. Bake the cupcakes for 15 minutes; then rotate the pan to ensure even baking and bake for another 15 minutes. After 30 minutes the cupcakes should have risen slightly and there should be some slight cracking patterns evident on their tops.

8. Remove the finished cupcakes from the oven and allow them to cool before frosting.

Sea Salt Brownies

Makes 9 to 12 Large Brownies

This recipe gives you one of the richest dessert choices on your diet. Offer this chocolatey, decadent dessert to guests, even those who love conventional treats.

- 1 pound cooked black beans
- 2 eggs, beaten
- 4 tablespoons butter, melted
- ¼ cup brewed espresso
- 1 teaspoon liquid stevia
- 1 teaspoon vanilla extract
- ¼ teaspoon salt
- 2 tablespoons almond flour
- ¼ teaspoon baking soda
- ½ cup cocoa powder
- Coarse sea salt for topping

1. Preheat the oven to 350°F. Purée the beans in a food processor until they reach a thick, soupy texture (more like cake batter than chicken broth).

2. Once the beans are puréed, add the eggs, butter, and espresso. Pulse these ingredients together to mix.

3. Add the stevia, vanilla, salt, almond flour, baking soda, and cocoa powder to the food processor. Let the food processor run until all ingredients are thoroughly incorporated. The color and texture should resemble chocolate cake mix: a rich, nutty brown with a light cocoa smell.

4. Bake in a greased pan that will produce the thickness that you prefer, 9 by 9 inches for thicker brownies or 9 by 13 inches for thinner, chewier brownies.

5. Bake at 350°F; the brownies need about 10 minutes for every ½ inch of thickness. Rotate the pan at the halfway mark to ensure the brownies are evenly baked.

6. Test for doneness with a knife, but remember that it might not come out completely clean due to the chewy texture of the brownies.

7. Allow brownies to cool for at least 10 minutes before slicing. Sprinkle with coarse sea salt.

15

CLEANSING BEVERAGES

There's no substitute for staying hydrated when you're fighting candida overgrowth. But there are times when you want something different, and there are also times when you might want the special boost that a natural flush of your colon gives you.

Why should you cleanse at all? We put our colons through so much with the average modern lifestyle. Alcohol doesn't hit only your liver, and cigarettes aren't hurting only your lungs. Those trips through the drive-through stress not only your belly and your figure. All of these things, not to mention stress, ensure that the colon is under fire most of the time. Add candida overgrowth to all of that and the colon can't keep up.

The waste matter that gets backed up in your colon can actually help candida breed and thrive, so colonic flushing can help you fight it. Since hardened fecal matter can cling to the inside of your intestines and colon for a very long time, colonics can help your dietary change work much more quickly. This is going to be especially helpful to those who suffer from chronic constipation.

The risk that colonics carry with them is that you can also flush out beneficial bacteria when you flush your digestive system out. Therefore, they're really only for those for whom constipation is a major problem. Harsh flushing, such as the sea salt flushes that accompany the Master Cleanse, is too much for regular use in a candida cleanse regimen. Instead, stick to regular consumption of flaxseeds and other natural fibers, and add one of these drinks to your diet a few times a week.

In this chapter:

Liver Flush

Makes 1 Serving

It may not be the tastiest drink in the world, but it clears your livers of toxins and any other dangerous buildups associated with candida. You can do it once daily if you choose to.

- 1 cup water
- 1 tablespoon olive oil
- 1 clove garlic
- Small chunk of fresh ginger, peeled

Blend all the ingredients and drink quickly.

Ginger Tea

Makes About 2 Cups

Enjoy this immune-boosting tea as often as you like. And remember, you can make tea from almost any spice or root you enjoy.

- 1-inch piece of fresh ginger, peeled and grated
- 1 slice lemon
- 2 cups boiling water

Add ginger to boiling water. Continue to boil for 20 minutes. Strain and serve with a slice of lemon.

Avocado Cream Smoothie

Makes 1–2 Servings

If you haven't tried avocado in a sweet dish, you're missing out. This smoothie will make you a believer.

- 1 medium avocado, peeled and pitted
- 1 cup coconut milk
- Stevia to taste
- 6 ice cubes

Blend the avocado, coconut milk, stevia, and ice together until smooth.

Immune-Booster Juice

Makes 2 Servings

Juicing with vegetables can only help you rebuild your immune system. The antioxidants, enzymes, minerals, and vitamins that these foods are full of fight candida valiantly. You will see that these recipes tell you to use a blender rather than a juicer so you still get the benefits of all the fiber in the ingredients.

- Handful of spinach
- Handful of fresh herbs (cilantro, parsley, or basil)
- 1 celery stalk
- Juice of 1 lemon
- 1 clove garlic (optional)
- 2 glasses of water

Add all ingredients into the blender and process until smooth. Best very cold.

Coconut Milk

Makes About 4 Cups

On the candida regimen, coconut milk is a constant. Why not make your own? It's delicious, and you'll taste the difference.

- 2 cups unsweetened shredded coconut
- 4 cups water

- 1 teaspoon vanilla extract
- 6 drops stevia

---

1. Soak coconut in water for 1 to 2 hours (do not discard water).

2. In a high-speed blender, combine coconut, water, vanilla, and stevia and process on highest speed for several minutes.

3. Strain liquid through cheesecloth, discarding solids. Chill.

Delicious Creamy Almond Milk

Makes About 2 Cups

Just like coconut milk, almond milk is a must for candida sufferers. You'll be shocked at how much better it tastes freshly made, and you can sweeten it as much or as little as you like. In the mood for something different? You can add vanilla extract if you choose.

• ⅓ cup raw almonds	• 2 cups water

1. Soak almonds overnight, and then rub the skins off.

2. Put the almonds and water (2 cups fresh water, not the soaking water) in the blender and blend until pulverized. Strain the milk with a fine mesh strainer or cheesecloth. Chill. You may sweeten with stevia to taste if you like.

Green Goodness Juice

Makes 1 Serving

Water is the perfect drink for everyone. But every once in a while you need a change, and this juice is the perfect way to do it.

- 2 packed cups baby spinach
- 1 cucumber (if using a juicer, unpeeled; if using a blender, peel)
- 1 celery stalk
- ½-inch piece of fresh ginger, peeled
- Juice of 1 lemon

Process using either a blender or juicer. Chill and serve.

Mixed Veggie Juice

Makes 1 Serving

This recipe is the V8 for candida sufferers. The difference is it is free of V8's many additives and preservatives, which attack the digestive system.

- 1 tomato
- 1 stalk celery, just the tender center stalk; trim and discard the tougher bottom
- ½ cup baby spinach leaves
- ½ cup fresh parsley

Process using either a blender or juicer. Chill and serve.

Avocado Apple Juice

Makes 2 Servings

Now that apples are back on your list, take advantage of it. You may not have considered teaming up apples and avocados, but the result is delicious and nutritious.

- 1 medium avocado
- 1 green apple, peeled and chopped
- Squeeze of fresh lemon or lime juice
- 1 cup water
- 2 mint sprigs

Blend everything except the mint on high speed until smooth. Serve with a sprig of mint on top.

Green Juice

Makes 2 Servings

This juice is absolutely packed with vitamins and minerals. It is also high in fiber.

- 4 cups kale, tough center stalks discarded, steamed
- ½ head collard greens (about 6 leaves)
- 1 English cucumber
- ½ bunch fresh parsley (about 1 cup lightly packed)
- ½ bunch fresh cilantro (about ½ cup lightly packed)
- Juice of ½ lemon

Process all except the lemon juice using either a blender or juicer. Add lemon juice after processing and mix well. Chill and serve. You can also omit lemon, and add yogurt and stevia for a smoothie.

16

SAUCES, DRESSINGS, AND EXTRAS

In a way, these recipes are the most fun. Even when you're really drag-
ging, these tasty sauces, dressings, and pick-me-ups can help keep
you committed to your candida cleanse and diet.

In this chapter:

Avocado Salad Dressing

Makes About 1 Cup

This dressing uses the natural creaminess of the avocado to create a rich, fabulous dressing. The best part? It takes minutes to make.

- 1 avocado
- 3 tablespoons olive oil
- 1 tablespoon fresh lemon juice
- ½ cup water
- ¼ teaspoon sea salt
- ¼ teaspoon black pepper

1. In a food processor or blender, purée avocado, olive oil, lemon juice, and water until smooth.

2. Season with salt and pepper to taste. Serve over green or chopped salads.

Caesar Dressing

Makes About ¾ Cup

This savory dressing is like no other. Don't be afraid to add an anchovy.

- 1 large clove garlic, crushed
- 1 teaspoon fresh lemon juice
- ¼ teaspoon dry mustard
- 1 anchovy fillet
- 1 whole egg
- ½ cup olive oil
- ¾ teaspoon salt
- ⅛ teaspoon black pepper

Combine all ingredients in a food processor or blender and process until smooth.

Tangy Dill Dressing

Makes About 1 Cup

This is probably one of the best dressings around, whether candida is an issue in your life or not. In fact, once you try it, you won't go back.

- ¼ cup olive oil
- ¼ cup water
- ¼ cup apple cider vinegar
- Several stalks fresh dill weed, to taste
- Mustard powder to taste
- Stevia to taste

- 1 tablespoon chopped red onion
- 2 cloves garlic
- ½ teaspoon Himalayan rock salt
- Several black olives (not prepared in vinegar)
- Black pepper to taste

Combine all ingredients in a food processor or blender and process until smooth.

Mayonnaise

Makes About 1 Cup

Making your own mayonnaise is far easier than you think, and chances are that once you've had your own homemade version you won't want the other kind again.

- 1 large egg yolk
- ½ teaspoon sea salt
- 1 teaspoon fresh lemon juice
- 1 teaspoon water
- ½ cup olive oil
- Dash of smoked paprika or any ground spices you like

1. Add egg yolk, salt, lemon juice, water, and any seasonings to a blender or food processor.

2. Blend well on medium-high speed. Slowly drizzle the oil into the egg mixture until you have added all of it, keeping the blender on medium-high speed the whole time. If you add the oil too quickly, the emulsion won't work and the mayonnaise will break up.

3. Blend until you have a creamy, opaque emulsion—mayonnaise. Keep refrigerated.

Green Goddess Dressing

Makes About 2 Cups
The origins of the name of this dressing are a mystery, but its continued popularity definitely isn't. Mild yet flavorful, this dressing will be one of your favorites.

- 1 avocado
- 2 tablespoons olive oil
- 1 tablespoon apple cider vinegar
- 1 tablespoon fresh lemon juice
- ½ teaspoon herbes de Provence
- ½ teaspoon sea salt
- 3 to 5 drops liquid stevia
- 1 cup water

Combine all ingredients in a food processor or blender and process until smooth.

Herb Gravy

Makes About 1 Quart

Never waste your pan drippings. Instead, make gravy and improve all your recipes.

- 1 quart chicken stock
- 2 medium onions, coarsely chopped
- 2 cloves garlic
- Pan drippings from a roasted chicken or turkey
- ½ teaspoon sea salt
- 1 tablespoon chopped fresh thyme

---

1. In a medium saucepan, bring chicken stock, onions, and garlic to a boil. Reduce heat and simmer until onions and garlic are soft, about 30 minutes.

2. Pour pan drippings into saucepan. Blend mixture in a food processor or blender until smooth.

3. Place mixture back in saucepan and reheat; then season with salt and thyme. Serve over turkey, mashed cauliflower, or anything else.

Avocado Pesto

Makes About 1 Cup

How does a richer, creamier version of pesto sauce—one that won't bother your candida—sound?

- 3 teaspoons pine nuts
- 3 teaspoons chopped walnuts
- Leaves from 1 large bunch fresh basil
- 1 large avocado, mashed
- 3 teaspoons olive oil
- 3 large cloves garlic
- Zest of 1 lemon
- Sea salt and black pepper to taste

1. Pulse nuts and basil in a food processor until finely ground.

2. Add other ingredients to nut mixture and process until smooth. Adjust seasonings and serve.

Kale Pesto Sauce

Makes About 1 Cup

What happens when kale is the source of green in your pesto? A sauce that takes health and taste to the next level.

- 1 (6 to 8-ounce) bunch kale, tough stems removed, steamed until bright green
- ½ cup toasted almonds
- 4 cloves roasted garlic
- ½ teaspoon sea salt or more to taste
- 2 tablespoons fresh lemon juice
- 1 tablespoon olive oil
- Pinch of red pepper flakes

1. Pulse kale in a food processor until chopped. Add almonds and garlic and pulse to incorporate.

2. Add salt, lemon juice, oil, and pepper flakes. Continue pulsing until pesto reaches desired consistency.

Breakfast Seasoning

It's wonderful to mix up your own favorite seasoning blends in advance—another great time saver and a fantastic way to get things tasting just the way you love them.

- 1 tablespoon smoked paprika
- ½ teaspoon sea salt
- 1 tablespoon garlic powder
- 1 teaspoon black pepper
- 1 teaspoon onion powder
- Pinch of cayenne pepper
- 2 teaspoons dried oregano
- ½ teaspoon dried ground sage
- 1 teaspoon dried thyme

Combine all ingredients and store in airtight container.

Ranch Dressing

Makes About 1½ Cups

Dipping everything from carrots to fries in ranch dressing is as American as apple pie. No candida-free lifestyle is complete without this dressing.

- ½ cup nondairy milk of your choice
- ½ cup Greek yogurt
- ¼ cup raw, unsalted sunflower seeds
- ¼ cup fresh lemon juice
- 1 tablespoon chia seeds
- 2 teaspoons dehydrated onion
- 1 teaspoon coconut aminos
- ½ teaspoon mustard powder
- 1 clove garlic
- ¼ teaspoon celery seed
- 1 tablespoon dried chives
- 1 tablespoon finely diced fresh parsley

1. Blend all ingredients except chives and parsley in a food processor or blender on high for 2 minutes, or until smooth.

2. Transfer to a resealable jar and stir in chives and parsley. Cover and refrigerate overnight before using.

Leek Coulis

Makes About 2 Cups

Don't be afraid of the fancy name—it's just a sauce. And it's great on just about everything, especially fish.

- ½ cup olive oil, divided
- 2 leeks, the white part and two inches of the green part, finely chopped
- 1 fennel bulb, finely chopped

- 1 tablespoon finely chopped fresh thyme
- 3 cups roughly chopped baby spinach
- 1 cup coconut milk
- ¼ cup fresh lemon juice
- ¼ teaspoon sea salt

1. Heat ¼ cup olive oil in a large, deep skillet. Sauté leeks and fennel until soft.

2. Stir in thyme and spinach and cook, covered, for 2 to 3 minutes, or until spinach is thoroughly wilted. Stir coconut milk into mixture.

3. Transfer mixture to a food processor or blender and purée on high until smooth. Blend in lemon juice and salt.

4. While processor is running on medium speed, slowly drizzle in the remaining ¼ cup olive oil until a smooth emulsion is formed. Serve over salmon or veggies.

Sweet Potato and Curry Marinade

Makes About 3 Cups

Don't be fooled by the very specific-sounding name of this recipe. You will rarely find a more versatile sauce than this one, which ranges from marinade to dip in no time and goes beautifully with almost anything.

- 1 medium sweet potato, cubed
- ½ cup sliced red onion
- 2 cloves garlic
- 1 tablespoon grape seed oil
- 1 cup coconut milk
- 2 tablespoons fresh lemon juice
- 1 tablespoon curry powder
- ⅛ teaspoon sea salt
- 2 tablespoons tightly packed finely chopped fresh cilantro
- 1 teaspoon tightly packed finely chopped fresh mint

1. Preheat oven to 400° F and set aside a small baking sheet lined with parchment paper.

2. Put cubed sweet potato, sliced red onion, garlic, and oil on the baking sheet and mix with your hands until everything is combined very well. Roast for 20 minutes, or until sweet potatoes are very tender. Remove from oven and allow to cool for several minutes.

3. In a food processor or blender combine coconut milk, water, lemon juice, curry powder, salt, and roasted vegetables, and process on high for 2 minutes, or until smooth.

4. Pour mixture into a bowl and stir in fresh herbs. Allow to cool completely and use as a salad dressing, sauce, dip, or marinade.

5. To use as a marinade, add to a resealable plastic bag along with meats and marinate overnight in the refrigerator.

Yogurt Cheese

Makes 1¼ Cups Cheese

This cheese is absolutely fantastic. It is easy to make and absolutely safe and healthy for the candida-free diet.

- 1 quart Greek yogurt
- 3 tablespoons finely chopped fresh chives
- 2 tablespoons chopped fresh flat-leaf parsley
- ½ teaspoon minced garlic
- ¾ teaspoon sea salt
- ⅛ teaspoon white pepper or to taste

1. Fold a large piece of cheesecloth twice to form a four-layer, roughly 18-inch square. Place in a sieve set over a large bowl, and spoon yogurt into center. Gather the four corners and tie a piece of kitchen twine just above the yogurt to form a tight bundle.

2. Let yogurt (still in the sieve over a bowl) drain in refrigerator at least 8 hours and up to 24 hours.

3. Cut open cheesecloth. Transfer yogurt cheese to a bowl. Stir chives, parsley, garlic, salt, and pepper into yogurt cheese. Serve and enjoy.

Sweet Almond Sauce

Makes ½ Cup

This is one of those basics that you'll want to keep around—and it takes just minutes to make.

- ¼ cup almond butter (or nut butter of your choice)
- ¼ cup almond milk (or nut milk of your choice)
- 5 drops stevia
- ¼ teaspoon ground cinnamon
- Pinch of ground cardamom
- ½ teaspoon carob powder

1. Place all ingredients in a blender or food processor and blend until smooth. Add more milk if necessary to reach desired consistency.

2. Pour over warm sweet potato rounds or pancakes.

Basic Candida-Safe Bread

Makes 1 Loaf

This basic bread is absolutely delicious and can be your go-to for everything from sandwiches to French toast to anything else you're missing. Keep it on hand at all times.

- 2 cups flaxseed meal
- 1 cup almond flour
- 1 cup hazelnut flour
- ¼ cup whole flaxseeds
- ¼ cup sesame seeds
- 4 teaspoons baking soda
- ½ teaspoon sea salt
- ½ cup unsweetened almond milk
- 8 egg whites
- ¼ teaspoon liquid stevia (optional)

1. Preheat the oven to 375°F. Line a loaf pan lengthwise with a strip of parchment paper and grease the two sides of the pan that remain exposed.

2. In a large bowl, mix flours, flaxseeds, sesame seeds, baking soda, and salt.

3. In a separate bowl, whisk together almond milk, egg whites, and liquid stevia.

4. Add the wet ingredients to the dry ingredients and stir. You should have a thick, sticky batter with no lumps. Pour the bread batter into the greased and lined loaf pan.

5. Bake for 45 minutes; then rotate the pan and bake for another 35 or 45 minutes. The baked bread should be golden and crisp on the top, but springy when pressed.

6. Let the bread cool for at least 5 minutes before you remove it from the pan, and then at least another 15 minutes before you slice it.

Buckwheat Tortillas

Makes 3–4

You haven't made tortillas before? No problem. It's easy, and these don't involve lard.

- 1¼ cups buckwheat flour, divided
- ¼ teaspoon sea salt
- ½ cup water, at room temperature
- ½ teaspoon olive oil

---

1. Mix 1 cup flour with the salt and make a well in the center. Put the oil and water in the well. Stir well with a fork until it forms a dough and clumps together in a ball.

2. Preheat a pan—cast iron is best—with no oil. Sprinkle some of the remaining flour on a work surface, take a golf-ball-sized piece of dough, and flatten it with your hand.

3. Keep turning it over, making sure it is well-floured each time. Roll it out with a rolling pin if you like. Make it as thin as a tortilla, but be careful not to make it too big. Cook on the hot pan for about 3 minutes on each side.

INDEX

Made in the USA
San Bernardino, CA
31 March 2016